The Lost Bible of Herbal Medicine & Natural Remedies

Unlocking Nature's Healing Power with the Ultimate Collection of Medicinal Herbs and Ancient Step-by-Step Recipes for Today's Health

TABLE OF CONTENTS

INTRODUCTION

Herbal medicine encompasses the utilization of medicinal plants to prevent and alleviate ailments, ranging from age-old traditional remedies to standardized herbal extracts (Firenzuoli & Gori, 2007). These remedies, rooted in cultural beliefs and personal experiences, span across diverse regions globally, offering a spectrum of effects, from invigorating brews to concentrated herbal formulations. Unlike conventional drugs, herbal medicines, which can encompass plant parts, vitamins, or minerals, are not bound by premarketing safety and efficacy regulations (Mamtani et al., 2015).

According to the World Health Organization (WHO), herbal medicine encompasses herbs, herbal materials, and preparations derived from plant components, serving as active ingredients in various formulations (World Health Organization, 2000). These components, sourced from leaves, stems, flowers, roots, and seeds, form the basis of herbal remedies utilized worldwide. Despite their widespread use, herbal medicines undergo less stringent regulatory scrutiny compared to conventional pharmaceuticals. This leniency has fueled a surge in herbal medicine adoption globally, with individuals turning to these products to address an array of health concerns across diverse healthcare settings (El-Dahiyat et al., 2020).

Natural Healing: The Holistic Approach to Wellness

Holistic healing embraces a comprehensive approach to health and wellness by considering the entirety of an individual, including physical, mental, emotional, and spiritual dimensions. This method stands in stark contrast to traditional medical practices that typically concentrate on treating specific ailments or symptoms, often overlooking the broader aspects of a person's existence. Holistic healing aims to achieve internal balance and foster overall well-being by integrating different facets of life.

A fundamental principle of holistic healing is the body's intrinsic capacity for self-healing. Supporting this natural capability involves creating an optimal environment for healing through various practices and therapies. These can range from nutritional guidance and physical activity to psychotherapy, spiritual counseling, and the use of natural remedies and preventive care to maintain health.

CHAPTER 1: FOUNDATIONS OF HERBAL HEALING

1.1 Introduction

Herbal medicine, tracing back to ancient times, stands as humanity's earliest healthcare practice, cherished across both developed and developing nations. In ancient societies, reliance on nature extended beyond sustenance and shelter to encompass medicinal solutions, with indigenous peoples discerning between beneficial herbs and potentially harmful ones. Presently, research underscores the medicinal potential of around 50,000 plant species (Msomi & Simelane, 2018), with pivotal drugs like aspirin, morphine, digitoxin, and quinine owing their origins to herbal sources validated through scientific inquiry (Wachtel-Galor & Benzie, 2011). This knowledge, passed down through generations, forms the bedrock of numerous traditional medical systems worldwide.

In contemporary times, herbal medicine remains the cornerstone of healthcare for roughly 80% of the global population, particularly prevalent in developing nations (World Health Organization, 2023). Moreover, industrialized countries like France and Germany witness a burgeoning trend in herbal prescriptions. Nonetheless, concerns persist regarding the safety of all herbal remedies (Msomi & Simelane, 2018). Over the centuries, traditional medicine has yielded invaluable insights into herb selection, preparation, and application. Upholding the same standards of rigorous clinical and scientific scrutiny ensures the efficacy and safety of these therapeutic interventions, positioning them as credible alternatives to Western medical practices.

1.2 Basic Principles of Herbal Medicine

The foundational principles of herbal medicine, based on recent research, are as follows:

Utilization of Medicinal Plants: Herbal medicine uses plant-based ingredients, including extracts and teas, recognized for their health benefits and therapeutic properties. These plants are sources of various chemical compounds that affect the body to prevent or treat diseases (Matole et al., 2021).

Integration with Traditional Systems: Traditional medicine boasts a rich heritage, rooted in the theories, customs, and observations of diverse cultures throughout history. These practices, often steeped in mystique and tradition, serve not only to maintain well-being but also to prevent, diagnose, manage, and treat illnesses (Firenzuoli & Gori, 2007). Within this framework, herbal medicine emerges as a cornerstone, intricately interwoven into the fabric of various traditional

6

healing systems. Its integration is deeply entrenched in longstanding cultural norms and beliefs, forming an essential component of holistic healthcare practices worldwide.

Complexity of Ingredients: Herbal medicines are composed not only of primary active ingredients but also of a range of secondary substances that interact to enhance therapeutic effects. These may include vitamins, minerals, and other bioactive compounds that facilitate the absorption and effectiveness of the main active principles (Capasso et al., 2003).

Challenges in Standardization: One of the major challenges in herbal medicine is the standardization and quality control of herbal products. Due to the complex nature of plant materials and variations in growing conditions, preparation, and preservation, achieving consistent quality and efficacy in herbal medicines is difficult. This impacts both their safety and effectiveness (Goldman, 2001).

Safety and Ethical Considerations: Ensuring the safety and ethical production of herbal medicines is paramount. This includes addressing ethical challenges across the supply chain, from cultivation and harvesting to clinical use. Herbal medicine must align with global values such as care, respect, honesty, and fairness to enhance its ethical standards and acceptance (Chatfield et al., 2018).

1.3 Benefits of Herbal Treatments over Conventional Medicine

Herbal treatments offer numerous benefits over conventional medicine, appealing to individuals seeking natural alternatives to pharmaceuticals. Grounded in the holistic principles of healing, these treatments emphasize prevention and the natural balance of the body, making them an attractive option for those interested in an organic lifestyle or cautious of synthetic additives. We now offer a comprehensive exploration of the many benefits of herbal remedies:

1.3.1. Holistic Healing

Herbal treatments often address the underlying problems rather than just alleviating symptoms. Many herbal therapies are designed to enhance the body's natural healing mechanisms, promoting overall wellness rather than merely treating specific ailments.

- *Nutritional Approaches*: Nutrition plays a critical role in holistic healing. The emphasis is on consuming whole, unprocessed foods that nourish the body and support its natural healing processes. Holistic nutritionists often recommend diets rich in organic fruits and vegetables, whole grains, lean proteins, and healthy fats, all of which provide essential nutrients and energy necessary for maintaining health and preventing disease. By addressing dietary deficiencies and promoting a balanced diet, holistic practitioners believe that nutrition can significantly affect one's health, mood, and energy levels.

- *Mind-Body Techniques*: Mind-body techniques are central to the holistic approach, emphasizing the powerful connection between physical health and mental well-being. Practices such as yoga, meditation, and tai chi are employed not only to improve physical fitness and flexibility but also to calm the mind, reduce stress, and enhance overall emotional resilience. These practices help individuals develop a deeper awareness of their bodies and the emotional states that affect their health, leading to greater self-care and symptom management.

- *Natural Remedies and Supplements*: While holistic healing often incorporates elements of conventional medicine, it also heavily utilizes natural remedies and supplements derived from plants and minerals. These natural products are used to boost the body's health and combat illness. Herbal remedies, essential oils, and homeopathic treatments are selected based on their ability to support the body's natural functions and promote healing. They are often preferred for their lower incidence of side effects compared to synthetic pharmaceuticals.

- *Preventive Health and Lifestyle Changes*: Prevention is a fundamental aspect of holistic healing. Holistic practitioners advocate for lifestyle changes that support health and prevent disease. This might include regular physical activity, adequate sleep, stress management techniques, and a healthy social life. By adjusting lifestyle factors that contribute to illness, holistic healing empowers individuals to take control of their health and maintain their wellness proactively.

- *Comprehensive Healing Techniques*: Holistic healing is inherently comprehensive, often blending various healing traditions and modern medical practices. This might involve combining acupuncture or massage therapy with conventional medical treatments to address both the symptoms and underlying causes of a condition. The goal is to use the best of both worlds to foster optimal health.

These holistic healing approaches aid in restoring body balance and preventing future health issues, aligning with many traditional health practices that focus on maintaining lifelong health. The use of complex herbal formulations in systems like Traditional Chinese Medicine customizes diagnosis and the choice of herbs to the specific symptoms and conditions of the patient, thereby increasing the efficacy of the treatment (Liu, 2010).

Natural Composition

Herbal treatments are derived from the seeds, berries, roots, leaves, bark, or flowers of plants for medicinal purposes. Unlike conventional medicines, which often contain synthetic chemicals, herbal remedies utilize natural components. This natural composition is perceived as gentler on the body, potentially reducing the risk of unwanted chemical side effects. This makes it appealing for those who prefer a more organic approach to healthcare.

Lower Side Effects

One of the significant benefits of herbal treatments is their lower incidence of side effects compared to conventional drugs. Although not devoid of risks, herbal medicines generally produce fewer adverse effects when used correctly. This is partly due to the less concentrated nature of the active ingredients in herbal remedies compared to those in synthetic drugs. Additionally, the holistic nature of herbs, containing multiple supportive constituents, can help mitigate the harsh effects of active ingredients.

Cost-Effectiveness

Herbal remedies can be more cost-effective than conventional medicines. Many herbs used in these treatments can be grown at home or purchased at a relatively low cost, making herbal treatments a valuable option for health management, especially in less affluent regions or among those looking to reduce healthcare expenses.

Support of Body Systems

Herbs often support entire body systems rather than just treating individual symptoms. For instance, some herbs are known for their ability to support the immune system, enhance digestion, or improve cardiovascular health. This systemic support is crucial for long-term health and is a cornerstone of preventive healthcare.

Integration with Other Natural Therapies

Herbal treatments can be easily combined with other natural therapies such as nutritional adjustments, physical therapies, and mind-body practices like yoga and meditation. This integration allows for a comprehensive approach to health that encompasses all aspects of an individual's lifestyle, enhancing the overall effectiveness of the healing process.

1.4 Techniques for Preparing and Using Herbs Effectively

Preparing and using herbs effectively involves several techniques that enhance their therapeutic properties and ensure their benefits are fully realized. Here is a quick overview of some common methods:

- *Infusions*: Infusions are one of the simplest ways to extract the active compounds from herbs, particularly from delicate parts like leaves and flowers. To prepare an infusion, pour boiling water over the herb and let it steep for about 10 to 15 minutes. This method is ideal for making herbal teas, which can be consumed to harness the healing properties of herbs.
- *Decoctions*: For tougher plant materials such as roots, bark, and seeds, decoctions provide a more effective extraction method. In this process, the herbs are boiled in water for a longer period, typically 20 to 30 minutes, allowing the hardy parts to release their active ingredients into the liquid.
- *Tinctures*: Tinctures involve soaking herbs in alcohol or a water-alcohol mixture for several weeks. This method extracts the active constituents effectively and preserves them for longer periods. Tinctures are taken in small doses and can be added to water or tea before consumption.
- *Topical Applications*: Herbs can also be used topically through salves, ointments, or oils. These are prepared by infusing herbs in a carrier oil or mixing them into a base like beeswax. Applied directly to the skin, these preparations can help with issues like inflammation, pain, and skin disorders.

1.5 Precautions and Safe Practices in Using Herbal Remedies

Herbal remedies offer numerous benefits, but like all forms of treatment, they must be used wisely to ensure safety and efficacy. The following are essential precautions and safe practices to keep in mind when using herbal remedies:

- *Consultation with Healthcare Providers*: Before starting any herbal treatment, it is crucial to consult a healthcare provider, especially for those with existing medical conditions or who

10

are taking other medications. Some herbs can interact with prescription drugs, potentially leading to adverse effects. A healthcare professional can provide guidance based on your health history and current treatments.

- Understanding Herbal Potency: Herbs can be potent, and their active compounds can have strong effects on the body (Passalacqua, Guarrera & De Fine, 2007). It is important to understand the potency of herbs and their expected impact. This awareness can prevent the misuse of herbs, which can lead to side effects such as allergic reactions, liver damage, or interference with other medications.

- *Accurate Dosage*: Following the correct dosage is vital. Just like conventional medicine, taking the right amount of herbal medicine is crucial for its effectiveness and safety. Overdosing can lead to complications while underdosing may render the treatment ineffective. Dosages can vary widely depending on the specific herb, the form in which it is taken, and the individual's health condition.

- *Quality and Purity of Herbs*: Only use high-quality, pure herbal products from reputable sources. The market for herbal remedies is not as tightly regulated as conventional medicine, which can lead to variations in the quality and concentration of herbal products. Using inferior-quality herbs can not only diminish the expected therapeutic effects but also pose serious health risks due to contaminants or pollutants.

- *Awareness of Side Effects*: While herbal remedies are generally safer than synthetic medications, they are not free from side effects. Users should be aware of possible adverse reactions and monitor their health closely after starting any herbal treatment. Common side effects might include gastrointestinal upset, headaches, or allergic reactions. If any severe or unexpected symptoms occur, discontinue use immediately and consult a healthcare provider.

- *Proper Storage*: Herbs should be stored properly to maintain their efficacy. Most herbs need to be kept in a cool, dry place away from sunlight, which can degrade their active ingredients. Some tinctures or infused oils may require refrigeration to prevent spoilage. Proper storage also prevents degradation and contamination of the herbs.

- *Educating Yourself*: Educating yourself about the herbs you plan to use is another essential safety measure. Understanding what each herb does, its benefits, potential side effects, and contraindications can help prevent harmful interactions and side effects. Reliable sources such as peer-reviewed journals, books by herbalists, and reputable websites can provide valuable information.

- *Long-Term Use and Monitoring*: Some herbal remedies may be intended for short-term use only, and long-term use could lead to complications. Continuous monitoring and periodic evaluations with a healthcare professional can help ensure that the use of herbal remedies does not inadvertently cause health issues.

If we adhere to these precautions and safe practices, we can safely enjoy the benefits of herbal remedies while minimizing potential risks. This responsible approach ensures that herbal treatments contribute to beneficial outcomes in holistic healing and health management.

CHAPTER 2: GLOBAL PERSPECTIVES ON HERBALISM: FROM ANCIENT WISDOM TO MODERN KEY FIGURES

2.1 Introduction

Herbalism has been a cornerstone of healing practices worldwide, blending ancient wisdom with modern applications. This chapter explores various herbal traditions, starting with Native American herbalism. It examines the history, practices, and remedies of herbalism, highlighting its deep roots in indigenous culture. The chapter then compares Native American herbalism with other traditional practices, such as Chinese and Ayurvedic medicine, emphasizing both similarities and unique distinctions. In the following section, the chapter provides an overview of influential herbalists like Barbara O'Neill, whose work has shaped contemporary herbal practices. Finally, the chapter discusses the philosophies underpinning these diverse practices and their contributions to modern herbalism, highlighting how these traditions continue to inform and evolve in contemporary health and wellness.

2.2 Native American Herbalism: History, Practices, and Remedies

Native American herbalism is steeped in a profound history that is intricately linked with the cultural practices and ways of life of different tribes throughout North America. This traditional form of herbalism has been transmitted across generations, showcasing the creativity and deep respect for nature that are hallmarks of these indigenous communities. The remedies and techniques developed are a testament to the rich herbal knowledge that has been cultivated and preserved over time.

2.2.1. Historical Context

The history of Native American herbalism spans centuries, tracing its roots to a time when tribes relied heavily on their immediate natural surroundings for sustenance and medicine. The knowledge of herbal remedies and medicinal plants was an integral part of Native American cultures, often preserved and communicated through oral tradition. This knowledge was considered a sacred trust, handed down from elders to younger members of the tribe, ensuring the continuation of practices that supported the health and well-being of their people (Ward, 2023).

Different tribes developed unique relationships with the plants around them, adapting their herbal practices to their specific environments. The Navajo, for instance, living in the arid southwestern

United States, cultivated knowledge of plants like sagebrush and yucca, which had medicinal properties suited to their desert climate. In contrast, the Iroquois of the northeastern United States had access to a more temperate climate, allowing them to use plants such as echinacea and wild ginger.

2.2.2. Practices:

The practices of Native American herbalism are characterized by a holistic approach to health and well-being, emphasizing balance between mind, body, and spirit. This approach is evident in the rituals and methods employed by different tribes.

- *Harvesting and Preparation*: One fundamental practice in Native American herbalism is the respectful harvesting and preparation of plants. Many tribes have traditional rituals to ask permission from the plant before harvesting it, expressing gratitude for its sacrifice (Ward, 2023). This spiritual dimension underscores the respect Native American cultures have for the natural world.

  The preparation of plants for medicinal purposes is meticulously carried out, with techniques varying based on the plant in question and its intended medicinal use. Common methods include creating teas, poultices, tinctures, and infusions. For instance, the Cherokee have traditionally used an infusion made from black cohosh roots to address women's health issues. Similarly, the Navajo have used poultices made from sagebrush leaves, which are applied as a moist mass to the body to alleviate joint pain and reduce inflammation.

- *Healing Ceremonies*: Another key aspect of Native American herbalism is the integration of herbal remedies into healing ceremonies. These ceremonies often combine herbal medicines with other spiritual practices, including chanting, drumming, and smudging (the burning of sacred herbs to cleanse the environment). The use of sage, cedar, and sweetgrass in smudging ceremonies is common across many tribes and is believed to purify the air and ward off negative energies.

- *Remedies*: Native American herbalism encompasses a wide variety of remedies tailored to address a range of ailments. The remedies draw on a deep understanding of the medicinal properties of different plants, many of which have been validated by modern science. Examples

14

include sage, echinacea, willow bark, yarrow, juniper, goldenseal, and elderberry (Mehl-Madrona, 2003; Ward, 2023).

a) *Sage*: One of the most significant plants in Native American herbalism is sage. Used both in ceremonies and as a medicinal herb, sage has antimicrobial and anti-inflammatory properties. Sage is used by the Navajo to address respiratory issues; they prepare it as a tea to help alleviate coughs and congestion.

b) *Echinacea*: The echinacea plant, also known as coneflower, is another staple in Native American herbalism. The Plains tribes, including the Sioux, have long utilized echinacea to boost the immune system and fight off infections. This practice has been supported by modern research, which shows that echinacea can stimulate the body's immune response (Nicolussi et al., 2022).

c) *Willow Bark*: Willow bark is a traditional remedy used by many tribes to alleviate pain and reduce fever. The Iroquois, for instance, brewed tea from willow bark to treat headaches and other ailments. Willow bark is effective in alleviating pain due to its content of salicin, a compound that is chemically similar to aspirin.

e) *Yarrow*: Yarrow is another common plant in Native American herbalism, known for its anti-inflammatory and wound-healing properties. The Cherokee used yarrow to treat cuts and bruises, creating poultices from its leaves to apply directly to the skin. Yarrow's ability to aid in blood clotting and reduce inflammation has been corroborated by modern studies.

f) *Juniper*: The juniper plant has been employed by various tribes for its antiseptic and diuretic properties. The Navajo used juniper berries to create a tea that served as a diuretic, helping to cleanse the body and support kidney health. Additionally, juniper oil has been used to treat skin conditions, highlighting its versatility in Native American herbalism.

g) *Goldenseal*: Goldenseal, another plant with deep roots in Native American herbal practices, has been used by tribes such as the Cherokee to treat digestive issues and infections. The plant contains berberine, a compound with antimicrobial properties, making it effective against various bacterial and fungal infections.

h) *Elderberry*: The elderberry plant has been a valuable remedy in Native American herbalism, particularly for its immune-boosting properties. Tribes like the Iroquois have used elderberry to create syrups and teas that help alleviate cold and flu symptoms. Recent research has supported these uses, demonstrating elderberry's antiviral and immune-stimulating effects (Mocanu & Amariei, 2022).

2.3 Comparisons with other Traditional Herbal Practices

Traditional herbal practices have been pivotal in healthcare across various cultures, with Native American herbalism, Chinese herbal medicine, Ayurveda, and other regional herbal traditions offering unique and effective remedies. This comparison aims to explore the differences and similarities among these practices, emphasizing their unique contributions to health and wellness.

Native American Herbalism

Native American herbalism has deep roots in the indigenous cultures of North America, encompassing diverse medicinal plants and holistic healing practices. Here's a look at its distinctive features:

- *Preparation Methods*: Native American herbalists prepare remedies in diverse ways, including infusions, decoctions, poultices, and salves, often in conjunction with rituals or prayers to enhance their efficacy.
- *Cultural Significance*: Healing practices often involve ceremonies, emphasizing the spiritual connection between humans and nature. Shamans or medicine men and women play central roles in healing communities, bridging the natural and spiritual worlds.

Chinese Herbal Medicine

Chinese herbal medicine, a key component of Traditional Chinese Medicine (TCM), boasts a practice history spanning thousands of years. It offers a unique framework for understanding health:

- *Yin-Yang Balance*: Chinese herbal medicine emphasizes balancing Yin and Yang energies in the body, aiming to maintain harmony and prevent illness.

- *Herbal Formulas*: TCM relies on complex herbal formulas, often composed of 4 to 12 ingredients. These formulas balance different properties, such as warming and cooling herbs, to target specific ailments.

- *Common Herbs*: Key herbs include ginseng, known for boosting vitality; licorice root, which harmonizes formulas and aids digestion; and astragalus, which supports the immune system.

- *Diagnosis and Customization*: Practitioners diagnose conditions through methods such as pulse reading and tongue inspection, customizing herbal treatments to individual patients.

Ayurveda

Ayurveda, originating around 6000 BC, is one of the oldest and most well-structured traditional healthcare systems in India, emphasizing prophylactic and therapeutic measures as its key components (Saggar et al., 2022). Ayurveda integrates herbal medicine with lifestyle practices:

- *Doshas*: Ayurveda classifies individuals into three doshas – Vata, Pitta, and Kapha – representing different bodily constitutions. Treatments aim to balance these doshas, utilizing diet, lifestyle, and herbs.

- *Herbal Treatments*: Common Ayurvedic herbs include turmeric, with anti-inflammatory properties; ashwagandha, which supports stress reduction; and triphala, a combination of three fruits aiding digestion.

- *Preparation*: Herbal remedies are prepared in various forms, including powders, capsules, decoctions, and oils, often combined with dietary recommendations to enhance effectiveness.

- *Integration*: Ayurveda's holistic approach encompasses mental, physical, and spiritual health, often integrating yoga and meditation into treatment plans.

African Herbalism

African herbalism encompasses diverse traditions across the continent, reflecting regional flora and cultural practices:

- *Traditional Healers*: African herbalism often relies on traditional healers or "sangomas," who use herbal remedies alongside spiritual practices.

- *Common Herbs*: Herbs such as Artemisia afra, used for respiratory conditions, and rooibos, known for its antioxidant properties, are staples in African herbalism.

- *Cultural Significance*: African herbalism is deeply intertwined with cultural practices, often involving rituals and ceremonies to address both physical and spiritual ailments.

- *Sustainability*: Herbalism in Africa places importance on sustainable harvesting and conservation of medicinal plants, recognizing their cultural and ecological significance (Ozioma & Chinwe, 2019).

Middle Eastern Herbalism

Middle Eastern herbalism draws from a rich history, influenced by Greek, Persian, and Islamic medicine:

- *Greek and Islamic Influence*: Middle Eastern herbalism has been shaped by ancient Greek medicine and Islamic scholars like Avicenna, whose texts integrated herbal remedies into medical practices.

- *Common Herbs*: Herbs such as cumin, known for aiding digestion; fenugreek, which helps regulate blood sugar; and licorice, with anti-inflammatory properties, are prevalent in Middle Eastern herbalism.

- *Unani Medicine*: Unani medicine, a prominent form of Middle Eastern herbalism, focuses on balancing bodily humors – blood, phlegm, yellow bile, and black bile – using herbal remedies.

- *Integration*: Middle Eastern herbalism often integrates dietary recommendations and lifestyle changes to complement herbal treatments, reflecting its holistic approach.

South American Herbalism

South American herbalism encompasses diverse traditions, heavily influenced by indigenous cultures and regional flora:

- *Indigenous Practices*: Indigenous cultures across South America, such as the Quechua and Mapuche, contribute significantly to the continent's herbal practices, integrating local plants into their healing traditions.

- *Common Herbs*: Herbs like coca leaf, used for its stimulant properties and pain relief; yerba mate, known for its antioxidant benefits; and cat's claw, which supports immune health, are staples in South American herbalism.

- *Cultural Significance*: Healing practices often involve shamanic rituals, emphasizing the spiritual connection between humans and nature, and blending herbal medicine with cultural traditions.

- *Preparation Methods*: Remedies are prepared as infusions, tinctures, or poultices, often in conjunction with spiritual rituals or prayers.

Tibetan Herbal Medicine

Tibetan herbal medicine, or Sowa Rigpa (science of healing), is a traditional healing practice influenced by Buddhist philosophy and Chinese medicine:

- *Mind-Body Connection*: Tibetan herbal medicine emphasizes the mind-body connection, aiming to balance the body's elements: wind, bile, and phlegm, through herbal remedies.

- *Common Herbs*: Herbs such as rhubarb root, used for digestive health; gentian, aiding liver function; and myrobalan, known for its antioxidant properties, are integral to Tibetan herbal medicine.

- *Herbal Formulas*: Tibetan medicine uses complex herbal formulas, often in the form of pills or powders, combining herbs to address specific ailments.

- *Integration*: Tibetan herbal medicine integrates herbal treatments with practices such as meditation, diet, and lifestyle changes, reflecting its holistic approach.

Japanese Herbalism

Japanese herbalism, or Kampo, has roots in traditional Chinese medicine, yet has developed its unique identity:

- *Chinese Influence*: Kampo draws from traditional Chinese medicine, adopting concepts such as Yin-Yang balance and herbal formulas, yet adapting them to Japanese culture.

- *Common Herbs*: Kampo includes herbs like Rehmannia glutinosa root, used for its anti-inflammatory properties; peony root, known for its calming effects; and licorice root, which harmonizes formulas and aids digestion.

- *Pharmaceutical Integration*: Kampo herbal formulas are integrated into modern Japanese healthcare, available through licensed pharmacists, reflecting its blend of traditional and modern medicine.

- *Diagnostic Methods*: Kampo relies on diagnostic methods such as pulse reading and patient interviews, customizing treatments to individual needs.

2.4 Contemporary Herbalism: Influential Herbalists and Their Philosophies

2.5.1. Barbara O'Neill

Barbara O'Neill, a prominent herbalist and naturopath, is known for her holistic approach to health and wellness. Her work has attracted significant attention in natural health circles, and she has influenced many through her teachings and writings.

O'Neill's practical approach to herbalism and natural health makes her teachings accessible to a broad audience. She focuses on common herbs and foods, offering guidance on integrating natural remedies into daily routines.

Philosophy:
O'Neill's comprehensive view of health encompasses the body, mind, and spirit. She stresses the importance of natural remedies and lifestyle changes, advocating for a balanced diet, proper exercise, and stress management. Her philosophy aligns with the holistic approach of traditional herbal practices, focusing on the interconnected aspects of health. Following are her philosophical principles:

- Natural Healing: O'Neill focuses on herbal remedies, nutrition, and lifestyle changes, believing in harnessing nature's healing power to support the body's innate ability to heal and restore balance.
- Holistic Approach: She views health as interconnected, advocating for addressing root causes with herbal remedies, diet, exercise, and mindfulness for overall well-being.
- Preventive Care and Self-Care: She promotes lifestyle modifications, including regular use of herbal remedies, to prevent illness and maintain long-term wellness.
- Accessible Herbalism: She educates her audience on integrating herbal remedies into daily routines, emphasizing practical applications for common ailments.

Contributions:
- *Literary Works*: O'Neill is an accomplished author, with publications on dietary recommendations, herbal treatments, and lifestyle changes that support well-being. Her bestselling book, "Self Heal By Design: The Role Of Microorganisms For Health," is a notable example. She has spoken at health conferences, covering topics from herbal remedies to lifestyle changes, making her insights accessible to a wide audience.
- *Educational Outreach:* O'Neill has contributed to herbal medicine through extensive educational programs, delivering numerous seminars and workshops on topics like nutrition, herbal remedies, and detoxification.
- *Community Engagement*: O'Neill's engagement in the natural health community has promoted holistic health practices. She collaborates with other practitioners and contributes to various publications, fostering a supportive network for those interested in herbal medicine and natural therapies.
- *Controversy and Challenges*: O'Neill's work has faced controversy. In 2019, she encountered regulatory challenges in Australia, which led to a ban on her practicing naturopathy and herbalism. This highlighted the complex regulatory landscape around natural health practices.

2.5.2. Rosemary Gladstar

Rosemary Gladstar, a distinguished herbalist and educator, is celebrated for her significant contributions to the field of herbal medicine. In 1978, she founded the California School of Herbal Studies, which was among the first herb schools in the United States. Additionally, she established both the International Herb Symposium and the New England Women's Herbal Conference. These events remain influential in advancing herbal education today.

Gladstar has been a strong advocate for sustainable herbalism, founding United Plant Savers (UpS), an organization dedicated to conserving medicinal plants. UpS promotes sustainable harvesting, supports local growers, and raises awareness about the ecological importance of medicinal plants, reflecting Gladstar's commitment to sustainability. With over four decades of experience, she has been influential in shaping modern herbal practices, making herbal remedies accessible to a broad audience.

Philosophy:

The philosophical principles of Gladstar are:

- Holistic Health: Gladstar's philosophy emphasizes a holistic approach to health, viewing the body, mind, and spirit as interconnected. She encourages the use of herbal remedies to support overall well-being, integrating them with other practices, such as mindfulness and diet, for comprehensive health.

- Accessible Herbalism: Gladstar advocates making herbal medicine accessible to everyone. She believes herbal remedies can be part of daily life, and her teachings demystify herbal practices, making them approachable and practical for beginners and seasoned herbalists alike.

- Nurturing and Intuitive: Gladstar's approach to herbal medicine emphasizes nurturing and intuition. She promotes the gentle, long-term use of herbs, recognizing their role in nourishing the body over time. This philosophy aligns with the Wise Woman Tradition, which emphasizes nurturing, self-care, and a connection to nature.

Contributions:

- *Literary Works*: Gladstar has authored several influential books, including "Herbal Healing for Women," "Rosemary Gladstar's Medicinal Herbs: A Beginner's Guide," and "The Science and Art of Herbalism." These works provide comprehensive guides to herbal medicine, covering topics from herbal identification to preparation and use, with a particular focus on women's health.

- *Educational Programs*: Besides the California School of Herbal Studies, Gladstar also established the Sage Mountain Herbal Retreat Center, where she offers workshops and courses. These programs provide hands-on experience in identifying, harvesting, and preparing herbs, fostering a practical understanding of herbal healing.

- *Community Engagement*: Gladstar has been actively involved in the herbal community, speaking at conferences, contributing to publications, and collaborating with other herbalists. This engagement has strengthened the herbal community and advanced the field of herbal medicine.

2.5.3. David Hoffmann

David Hoffmann is a prominent herbalist, educator, and author who has made significant contributions to the field of herbal medicine. Hoffmann has been a significant figure in herbal education, teaching herbal medicine at various institutions worldwide. His educational efforts include workshops, lectures, and courses, providing comprehensive knowledge about herbal practices to students and professionals alike.

Hoffmann has been involved in various professional organizations, including the American Herbalists Guild, where he served as a member of the advisory board. His involvement in these organizations has helped promote the integration of herbal medicine into mainstream healthcare, emphasizing the importance of herbal remedies in modern society. With decades of experience, Hoffmann's work has shaped modern herbal practices, blending traditional wisdom with scientific research.

Philosophy:
David Hoffmann's philosophy emphasizes:
- Holistic Health: Hoffmann views the body, mind, and spirit as interconnected. He believes in addressing the root causes of health issues, not just the symptoms, integrating herbal medicine with other holistic practices, such as nutrition, to support overall well-being.
- Scientific Integration: Hoffmann advocates for integrating herbal medicine with modern scientific research. He believes that traditional herbal knowledge and modern science can complement each other, helping to validate the therapeutic properties of herbs and advancing the field of herbal medicine.
- Herbal Education: Hoffmann is a strong proponent of herbal education, believing that knowledge is essential for empowering individuals to take control of their health. He

encourages people to learn about the properties and uses of herbs, making herbal medicine accessible to a wider audience.

- Practical Application: Hoffmann's philosophy emphasizes the practical application of herbal remedies, guiding individuals to incorporate herbs into their daily lives. He promotes the use of natural remedies, encouraging people to consider herbal medicine as part of a balanced approach to health.

Contributions:

- *Literary Works*: David Hoffmann has authored several influential books, including "Medical Herbalism: The Science and Practice of Herbal Medicine," This book, along with others such as "The Complete Illustrated Holistic Herbal," and "The Holistic Herbal: A Safe and Practical Guide to Making and Using Herbal Remedies", "The Herbal Handbook" and "An Herbal Guide to Stress Relief," has influenced countless practitioners and enthusiasts. These works provide comprehensive guides to herbal medicine, covering topics from herbal identification to preparation and use.

- *Educational Programs*: Hoffmann has taught at various herbal schools and institutions, including the California School of Herbal Studies and the National Institute of Medical Herbalists. His teachings cover a wide range of topics, from herbal identification to integrating herbal medicine into modern healthcare.

- *Clinical Practice*: Hoffmann has practiced as a clinical herbalist for many years, offering consultations that incorporate traditional herbal knowledge with modern science. His holistic approach allows him to tailor treatments to individual needs, providing comprehensive guidance to patients.

- *Community Engagement*: Hoffmann has been actively involved in the herbal community, speaking at conferences, contributing to publications, and collaborating with other herbalists. This engagement helps to strengthen the herbal community and promotes the integration of traditional and modern herbal medicine.

2.5.5. Susun Weed

Susun Weed is an influential herbalist, educator, and author known for her contributions to the field of herbal medicine. With over 50 years of experience, Weed's work has significantly impacted the herbal community, particularly through her focus on women's health and empowerment. Weed has been actively involved in mentoring aspiring herbalists, guiding them through the complexities of herbal medicine. She has also contributed to various herbal communities, fostering a supportive environment for those interested in herbal practices.

Philosophy:
Susun Weed has significantly influenced modern herbal practices through her teachings and philosophy.

- Wise Woman Tradition: Susun Weed's philosophy draws from this ancient approach to healing, emphasizing nurturing, intuition, and nature. It contrasts with clinical methods, promoting gentle, long-term herbal remedies for health support. Weed is a proponent of this holistic tradition, which integrates herbal remedies and lifestyle changes for well-being, especially in women, blending ancient wisdom with modern insights.
- Nourishing Herbs: Weed's philosophy promotes the use of nourishing herbs that can be incorporated into daily routines. She emphasizes plants that are safe for extended use, such as nettle and oat straw, and encourages herbal teas, infusions, and food-based remedies that can support holistic well-being over time.
- Holistic Health: Weed emphasizes the interconnection between the body, mind, and spirit, advocating for a holistic approach to health. Her teachings encompass not only herbal remedies but also lifestyle practices, such as diet and mindfulness, to achieve overall well-being.
- Women's Health: A key element of Weed's philosophy is a focus on women's health. She offers specialized guidance on herbs and practices that support women's wellness at different stages of life, from menstruation to menopause, recognizing the unique needs and cycles of the female body.

Contributions:
- *Literary Works*: Weed is an accomplished author, having written several influential books on herbal medicine. Her publications include "Wise Woman Herbal for the Childbearing Year," "The New Menopausal Years: The Wise Woman Way," "Healing Wise," and "Breast Cancer? Breast Health!" These books offer comprehensive guides to herbal remedies for women's health, covering topics such as reproductive health, pregnancy, and menopause.
- *Educational Programs*: Weed conducts various workshops and apprenticeships, sharing her knowledge of herbal medicine and the Wise Woman Tradition with learners. These programs

provide hands-on experience in identifying, harvesting, and preparing herbs, fostering a practical understanding of herbal healing.

- *Community Engagement*: Weed's work extends to the broader herbal community, where she contributes articles, gives talks at conferences, and collaborates with other herbalists. This engagement helps to strengthen the herbal community, promoting the integration of traditional and modern practices.

- *Supportive Networks*: Weed has helped create supportive networks for herbal enthusiasts, including the Wise Woman Forum, which provides a platform for individuals to share knowledge, experiences, and support. This community engagement has contributed to the growth and accessibility of herbal practices.

CHAPTER 3: ANTIOXIDANT-RICH HERBS AND RECIPES FOR BOOSTING IMMUNITY

3.1 <u>What Are Antioxidants</u>?

An antioxidant is a substance, whether it be a molecule, ion, or stable radical, that has the capability to inhibit or delay the oxidation process of other molecules. Put simply, antioxidants shield the body from harm inflicted by free radicals. Free radicals are molecules characterized by their instability due to unpaired electrons, rendering them exceptionally reactive. When these molecules interact with cellular elements like DNA, proteins, and lipids, they induce oxidative stress, culminating in cellular impairment, aging, and the onset of various diseases such as cancer, cardiovascular ailments, and neurodegenerative disorders.

3.1.2. Types of Antioxidants:

Antioxidants come in various forms, including vitamins, minerals, and phytochemicals:

Vitamin Antioxidants: Vitamins C and E are notable antioxidants. Vitamin C, a water-soluble vitamin, works in the cytoplasm and extracellular fluid, where it can donate electrons to free radicals. Vitamin E, a fat-soluble vitamin, works within the lipid membranes of cells, preventing oxidative damage to fatty acids.

Mineral Antioxidants: Minerals such as selenium and zinc are cofactors for antioxidant enzymes. These enzymes, including glutathione peroxidase and superoxide dismutase, play a critical role in reducing oxidative stress by catalyzing the conversion of harmful free radicals into harmless molecules.

Phytochemical Antioxidants: Plant-derived compounds such as polyphenols and carotenoids exhibit antioxidant properties. Polyphenols, found in foods like fruits, vegetables, and teas, can neutralize free radicals directly. Carotenoids, such as beta-carotene found in carrots, also act as antioxidants, and can be converted into vitamin A, further supporting the body's antioxidant defense mechanisms.

Synergistic Effects: Antioxidants can also work synergistically, enhancing each other's effects. For instance, vitamin C can regenerate oxidized vitamin E, allowing it to continue protecting cell membranes. This synergy helps to maintain a balanced antioxidant defense system, preventing oxidative stress from overwhelming the body.

3.1.3. The Role of Antioxidants in Preventing Oxidative Stress and Cellular Damage

The primary function of antioxidants is to neutralize free radicals by donating an electron, effectively stabilizing the radicals, and preventing further damage. In essence, antioxidants defend cells against the harmful effects of free radicals.

Oxidative stress arises from normal physiological processes and environmental interactions. A sophisticated network of antioxidants, both innate and dietary, helps protect cells from oxidative damage (Ogunro et al., 2023). Disruptions to this balance can lead to oxidative stress, contributing to various diseases, including gastrointestinal illnesses. Developing antioxidant therapies offers a promising avenue for treating such conditions, including inhibiting radical generation and promoting antioxidant activity.

3.1.4. Essential Antioxidants

Key antioxidants include nutrients like beta-carotene, lycopene, carotenoids, vitamins C and E, and compounds like thiols and ascorbic acid. Enzymes such as catalase, superoxide dismutase, and glutathione peroxidase play a crucial role in mitigating oxidative stress. Dietary antioxidants have been linked to health benefits, including reducing the risk of ailments like cancer and heart disease (Conti et al., 2016; Stanner & Weichselbaum, 2013). Plant-derived antioxidants, such as polyphenols, carotenoids, and vitamins, are of particular interest. However, evidence from supplementation studies with antioxidants like vitamin C, vitamin E, carotenoids, zinc, or selenium does not strongly support a reduction in disease risk (Conti et al., 2016; Kurutas, 2016; Ogunro et al., 2016).

3.2 Sources of Antioxidants

In order to fight diseases and enhance overall health, it's crucial to include foods rich in antioxidants in your diet. This section delves into a variety of antioxidant sources, including fruits, vegetables, beverages, and herbs. We'll examine their nutritional advantages and the roles they play in supporting a healthy body.

Fruits:

- Berries: Blueberries, strawberries, and raspberries are rich in antioxidants, including flavonoids, anthocyanins, and vitamin C. These powerful compounds aid in neutralizing free radicals and shielding the body from oxidative stress.
- Citrus Fruits: Oranges, lemons, and grapefruits contain high quantities of vitamin C, a powerful antioxidant. Vitamin C contributes to collagen production, supporting healthy skin and tissues.
- Pomegranates: Rich in polyphenols, including punicalagins and ellagic acid, pomegranates offer potent antioxidant properties that may reduce inflammation and oxidative stress.

Vegetables:
- Leafy Greens: Antioxidants such as vitamin C, beta-carotene, and lutein are plentiful in spinach, kale, and Swiss chard. They serve to safeguard cells from oxidative harm and promote the well-being of the eyes.
- Cruciferous Vegetables: Broccoli, Brussels sprouts, and cauliflower contain antioxidants such as sulforaphane and indole-3-carbinol, which contribute to detoxification and support cellular health.

Nuts and Seeds:
- Walnuts: These nuts are rich in polyphenols, including ellagic acid, and provide a source of vitamin E, which helps protect cell membranes from oxidative stress.
- Chia Seeds: Chia seeds are packed with antioxidants, including quercetin and chlorogenic acid, which may contribute to cardiovascular health by reducing inflammation.

Beverages:
- Green Tea: Green tea is rich in catechins, particularly epigallocatechin gallate (EGCG), a potent antioxidant that may reduce inflammation and support metabolism.
- Red Wine: In moderation, red wine offers antioxidants like resveratrol, which has been associated with cardiovascular benefits and anti-inflammatory properties.

Spices and Herbs:
- Turmeric: Turmeric boasts curcumin, a potent antioxidant renowned for its ability to alleviate inflammation and shield against oxidative harm.
- Cinnamon: Cinnamon is a rich source of polyphenols, including cinnamaldehyde, which has antioxidant properties that can aid in blood sugar regulation and metabolic health.

3.3 Overview of Herbal Sources Rich in Antioxidants

Herbs are a natural source of antioxidants, offering a range of compounds that help protect the body from oxidative damage. Incorporating herbs into the diet or as supplements can offer a range of antioxidant benefits, supporting overall health and helping to mitigate oxidative stress. Following are some herbal sources rich in antioxidants:

- Rosemary: Rosemary is packed with antioxidants, particularly rosmarinic acid and carnosic acid. These compounds contribute to its anti-inflammatory properties and may protect against oxidative damage to brain cells, supporting cognitive health. Rosemary can be used fresh or dried in a variety of dishes.

- Oregano boasts an array of antioxidants, including phenolic compounds like carvacrol and thymol, known for their antimicrobial attributes and potential in countering oxidative stress. It's a popular choice for enhancing the flavor of meats, pasta, and salads.

- Sage provides antioxidants such as rosmarinic acid and flavonoids, recognized for their anti-inflammatory and neuroprotective effects. Commonly used in culinary creations, sage adds complexity to both meat and vegetable dishes.

- Thyme is abundant in antioxidants, particularly phenolic compounds like thymol, acknowledged for their antimicrobial properties and potential to promote respiratory wellness. Frequently employed to season meats, soups, and stews, thyme adds aromatic depth to various dishes.

- Ginseng, a time-honored medicinal herb, derives from the root of the Panax ginseng plant. Renowned for its adaptogenic and antioxidant qualities, ginseng contains compounds such as ginsenosides and flavonoids. These antioxidants combat oxidative stress, bolstering vitality and cognitive function. Ginseng is commonly ingested in teas, capsules, or extracts.

- Ginkgo biloba offers a rich source of flavonoids and terpenoids, known for their antioxidant prowess. These compounds may fortify cognitive function and shield brain cells from oxidative damage. Typically consumed in supplement form, Ginkgo biloba is valued for its potential cognitive benefits.

- Milk Thistle: Milk thistle contains a potent antioxidant called silymarin, which has anti-inflammatory properties and supports liver health by protecting liver cells from oxidative stress. Milk thistle can be consumed as a supplement or as a tea.

- Ashwagandha: Ashwagandha is an adaptogenic herb that provides antioxidants such as withanolides. These compounds help reduce oxidative stress and support hormonal balance. Ashwagandha is typically consumed in supplement form or as a powder added to beverages.

- Mint: Mint is rich in antioxidants, featuring flavonoids such as luteolin and quercetin, renowned for their anti-inflammatory attributes and potential to combat oxidative stress. Whether infused in teas, tossed in salads, or garnishing desserts, mint adds a refreshing twist to culinary creations.

- Cilantro: Cilantro offers a plethora of antioxidants, including quercetin and vitamin C, prized for their anti-inflammatory effects and potential role in supporting detoxification processes. Fresh cilantro leaves are commonly incorporated into salads, salsas, and a diverse range of dishes, imparting a distinctive flavor and nutritional boost.

- Chamomile: Chamomile contains antioxidants such as apigenin and flavonoids, which contribute to its calming and anti-inflammatory properties. Chamomile tea is commonly used to promote relaxation and may support sleep quality.

3.4 Discussion on the Benefits of Antioxidant-Rich Herbs

Antioxidant-rich herbs are increasingly recognized for their numerous health benefits, providing a natural and effective means of combating oxidative stress and promoting overall well-being. The following discussion explores the key benefits of incorporating these herbs into one's diet, emphasizing their role in maintaining health and preventing disease.

- Herbs rich in antioxidants are crucial for protecting the body against oxidative stress, which occurs when there's an imbalance between free radicals and antioxidants in the body. Free radicals can damage cells, proteins, and DNA, contributing to a variety of health problems, including inflammation, aging, and chronic diseases. Herbs with high antioxidant content combat these free radicals, reducing oxidative stress and its harmful effects. This promotes cellular health and helps prevent diseases associated with oxidative stress, such as cardiovascular diseases, neurodegenerative disorders, and certain cancers.

- Additionally, antioxidant-rich herbs exhibit anti-inflammatory properties that complement their antioxidant prowess. Chronic inflammation is a significant contributor to diverse health problems, including arthritis, metabolic disorders, and even cancer. By quelling

31

inflammation, these herbs alleviate symptoms linked to chronic inflammatory conditions, bolster overall health, and potentially reduce the likelihood of developing associated ailments. This dual action—addressing both oxidative stress and inflammation—establishes a comprehensive approach to maintaining health.

- Moreover, these herbs can improve metabolic health. Antioxidant-rich herbs have been found to enhance insulin sensitivity, regulate blood sugar levels, and improve lipid profiles, making them valuable for managing diabetes and cardiovascular health. Regular consumption of these herbs can help reduce the risk of developing metabolic disorders, contributing to better overall health.

- Another notable benefit of antioxidant-rich herbs is their neuroprotective effects. Oxidative stress and inflammation are known to contribute to cognitive decline and neurodegenerative disorders such as Alzheimer's and Parkinson's disease. The antioxidants in these herbs can protect brain cells from damage, slow cognitive decline, and support healthy brain function. This makes them a valuable addition to the diet, particularly for those at risk of or experiencing cognitive decline.

- Lastly, incorporating antioxidant-rich herbs into daily meals is a simple yet effective way to promote better health. They can be used in cooking, teas, or supplements, making them accessible to a wide range of individuals. This accessibility, coupled with their diverse health benefits, makes these herbs an essential part of a healthy lifestyle.

3.5 Antioxidant-Rich Herbs

3.5.1. Turmeric: Curcumin as an antioxidant powerhouse.

Turmeric, a golden-yellow spice, is a culinary staple and medicinal herb with profound health benefits. Its primary active compound, curcumin, is a potent antioxidant that offers a range of therapeutic properties. Let's delve into turmeric's dual role as an herb and an antioxidant powerhouse.

Curcumin as an Antioxidant Powerhouse:

Curcumin stands out as the key compound in turmeric, boasting powerful antioxidant properties. Its antioxidant action directly neutralizes free radicals, preventing cellular damage and reducing oxidative stress, which contributes to aging and various health conditions. Curcumin also boosts the body's own antioxidant enzymes, amplifying its protective effects. These actions help lower the risk of conditions such as arthritis, neurodegenerative disorders, and certain cancers.

Anti-inflammatory Properties:

Turmeric's health benefits are further enhanced by its anti-inflammatory effects. Chronic inflammation is a major contributor to numerous health problems, including metabolic disorders, cardiovascular diseases, and cancer. Curcumin's ability to reduce inflammation complements its antioxidant effects, helping prevent and manage a variety of health conditions.

Turmeric and Medicinal Properties:

Turmeric's medicinal properties stem from its curcuminoid compounds, with curcumin being the most significant. It has been used in traditional medicine for thousands of years, particularly in India, for its ability to address various ailments. Scientific research has supported these traditional uses, showing curcumin's potential to protect against heart disease, Alzheimer's, and cancer, among other benefits (Sharifi-Rad et al., 2020).

Turmeric's Bioavailability and Consumption:

A significant hurdle in the therapeutic use of turmeric is the low bioavailability of curcumin. To address this, combining turmeric with black pepper, which contains piperine, significantly boosts the absorption of curcumin—by as much as 2,000%. Furthermore, because curcumin is fat-soluble, consuming it with a fatty meal enhances its uptake. This is the reason why many curcumin supplements are formulated with piperine and are advised to be taken alongside meals.

Benefits for Metabolic Health:

Turmeric's curcumin has been shown to improve metabolic health by regulating blood sugar levels and lipid profiles. This can aid in managing diabetes and cardiovascular health, making turmeric a valuable addition to a balanced diet.

Neuroprotective Effects:

Curcumin's role in enhancing brain-derived neurotrophic factor (BDNF) is particularly significant, supporting cognitive functions and aiding in the prevention of neurodegenerative diseases such as Alzheimer's. The increase in BDNF levels brought about by curcumin can also enhance memory and attention, underscoring the neuroprotective capabilities of turmeric.

3.5.2. Green Tea: Catechins and their Health Benefits

Green tea, derived from the leaves of the Camellia sinensis plant, has been enjoyed for centuries as a beverage and medicinal herb. It is particularly known for its potent antioxidant properties, largely attributed to its polyphenols, especially catechins (Musial, Kuban-Jankowska & Gorska-Ponikowska, 2020). The benefits of green tea, especially its antioxidant capabilities, are emphasized below.

Catechins and Antioxidant Activity:

Catechins, a type of polyphenol, are the primary compounds responsible for green tea's antioxidant effects. One key catechin, Epigallocatechin gallate (EGCG), is especially effective at neutralizing free radicals. Free radicals are unstable molecules that can damage cells, proteins, and DNA, leading to various health issues (Musial et al. 2022). By neutralizing these molecules, EGCG helps protect cells, reducing oxidative stress and potentially preventing chronic diseases such as cancer and cardiovascular ailments.

Anti-inflammatory Effects:

The anti-inflammatory properties of catechins found in green tea contribute significantly to its health benefits. Inflammation plays a pivotal role in numerous health conditions, ranging from arthritis to heart disease and cancer. By reducing inflammation, green tea has the potential to mitigate the risks associated with these conditions, offering a holistic approach to maintaining health.

Metabolic Health and Weight Management:

Consistent intake of green tea has been linked to enhanced metabolic well-being. Catechins, notably EGCG, have shown promise in regulating blood sugar levels, lipid profiles, and insulin sensitivity, offering potential benefits in managing diabetes. Moreover, green tea's ability to boost metabolism may support weight management, rendering it a beneficial component of a well-rounded diet.

Types of Green Tea and Production Process:

Green tea is available in various types, with differences in taste, caffeine content, and antioxidant properties. Sencha, for example, is a popular type grown in Japan, while other varieties include Bancha, Matcha, and Gyokuro. The technological process plays a significant role in green tea's antioxidant content. Unfermented green tea retains a higher concentration of catechins than black tea, which undergoes fermentation, transforming catechins into other compounds.

Health-Promoting Properties:

Green tea's health benefits extend beyond its antioxidant and anti-inflammatory effects. Research suggests that its polyphenols can help prevent various cancers, including lung, stomach, and prostate cancers, by inhibiting cancer cell growth and promoting cancer cell death without affecting healthy cells (Trisha et al., 2022). This makes green tea a potential adjunct to cancer prevention and treatment, though it should not replace medical therapy.

Bioavailability and Absorption:

To maximize the health benefits of green tea, we have to take in consideration its bioavailability. Green tea's catechins can be poorly absorbed into the bloodstream. To improve absorption, green tea can be paired with black pepper, which contains piperine, or taken with a fatty meal, enhancing the uptake of these beneficial compounds.

3.5.3. Ginseng: Saponins and immune-boosting properties.

Ginseng is notable for its antioxidant, anti-inflammatory, and immune-boosting properties, contributing to its status as a panacea in traditional medicine. The benefits and mechanisms of ginseng are discussed below.

Bioactive Components:

Ginseng's medicinal properties are attributed to its bioactive components, particularly ginsenosides. Ginsenosides are saponins, compounds that contribute significantly to ginseng's therapeutic effects. Nearly 50 types of ginsenosides have been identified in Panax ginseng root, with additional varieties found in other ginseng species, including American ginseng and Japanese ginseng (Schreiner et al., 2022).

Antioxidant Properties:

Ginseng serves as a potent antioxidant, countering the harmful effects of free radicals in the body. These unstable molecules have the potential to harm cells, proteins, and DNA, which can contribute to a variety of health problems including inflammation, aging, and chronic illnesses. The ginsenosides and additional compounds found in ginseng help mitigate oxidative stress, thereby safeguarding cells and enhancing overall health.

Anti-inflammatory and Immune-Boosting Effects:
Ginseng's anti-inflammatory properties complement its antioxidant effects, helping to alleviate inflammation-related conditions such as arthritis and cardiovascular diseases. Additionally, ginseng is known to boost immune function, enhancing the body's ability to fight off infections and other illnesses. This makes it valuable for promoting general health and preventing disease.

Central Nervous System Benefits:
Ginseng has a positive impact on the central nervous system (CNS), supporting brain function and reducing stress. Its neuroprotective effects help prevent cognitive decline and neurodegenerative disorders such as Alzheimer's disease. Additionally, ginseng has been shown to improve memory and learning, making it beneficial for maintaining cognitive function, particularly in older individuals.

Anti-cancer and Anti-diabetes Properties:
Ginsenosides in ginseng have also properties that may inhibit cancer cell growth and spread, offering potential anti-cancer benefits. Additionally, ginseng's impact on metabolic health can aid in regulating blood sugar levels, making it an effective tool for managing diabetes and minimizing its associated complications.

Cultural Significance and Modern Use:
Ginseng has been a staple in East Asian traditional medicine for over 2000 years, particularly in China, Korea, and Japan. Its popularity has since spread to Western countries, with ginseng being widely used in North America and Europe. The plant's name, Panax, means "cure for all," reflecting its diverse therapeutic potential.

3.5.4. Rosemary: Carnosic Acid and its Role in Protecting Neural Cells

Rosemary, an aromatic herb from the Lamiaceae family, is not only a culinary delight but also a powerful medicinal plant. The way in which rosemary functions as an herb and an antioxidant is highlighted below.

Bioactive Properties:

Extracts from rosemary are rich in bioactive substances such as phenolic compounds, including carnosic acid and carnosol (Nieto, Ros & Castillo, 2018). These elements are responsible for rosemary's antioxidant, anti-inflammatory, and antibacterial effects, rendering it an effective natural treatment and preservative for foods.

Carnosic Acid and its role in Protecting Neural Cells:

The compound carnosic acid, found abundantly in rosemary, serves as a vital guardian for neural cells. Functioning as an potent antioxidant, it effectively counters free radicals, which pose a threat to brain cells and are implicated in cognitive deterioration and neurodegenerative ailments such as Alzheimer's disease. By exerting neuroprotective properties, carnosic acid contributes to the preservation of brain health, enhancement of cognitive capabilities, and potentially diminishes the likelihood of age-related neurodegenerative disorders.

Food Preservation and Safety:

Rosemary's antioxidant and antimicrobial properties make it a valuable natural preservative. In food production, rosemary extracts help prevent oxidation, extending shelf life and reducing microbial contamination. This aligns with the growing demand for "clean label products," where natural preservatives are preferred over synthetic additives. The European Food Safety Authority (EFSA) has approved the use of rosemary extracts in food and beverages, allowing up to 400 mg/kg of carnosic acid and carnosol combined.

Health Benefits and Applications:

Beyond its neuroprotective and preservative properties, rosemary offers several health benefits:
- Hepatoprotective: Rosemary's bioactive compounds contribute to liver health, helping to protect against liver damage and supporting detoxification.
- Anti-inflammatory: The phenolic compounds in rosemary help reduce inflammation, which can alleviate conditions like arthritis and cardiovascular disease.

- Antioxidant: The phenolic compounds found in rosemary function as antioxidants, safeguarding cells from oxidative stress and lowering the risk of several chronic diseases.

Preparation and Extraction:

The method of extracting rosemary's bioactive compounds is crucial to its antioxidant properties. Various methods are used, including solvent extraction with oils, organic solvents, or mechanical pressing. Modern extraction techniques also include molecular distillation, which separates rosemary's antioxidant components efficiently.

3.5.5. Oregano: The Herb and Antioxidant for Neural Health

Oregano is a versatile herb known for its culinary use and medicinal properties. It consists of various plants from different families, notably the Verbenaceae and Lamiaceae families. It is established that oregano protects neural cells and functions as an antioxidant (Gutiérrez-Grijalva et al., 2018)

Phytochemicals and Their Functions:

Oregano's health benefits come from its phytochemicals, which are compounds derived from the secondary metabolism of plants. These compounds, which include essential oils and phenolic compounds, serve as a defense mechanism for plants against pathogens, pests, and environmental stressors. In humans, they offer several medicinal benefits.

Antioxidant Properties:

Oregano's phenolic compounds, including flavonoids and phenolic acids, demonstrate potent antioxidant capabilities (Gutiérrez-Grijalva et al., 2018). These antioxidants play a critical role in neutralizing free radicals, which are unstable molecules capable of causing harm to cells, proteins, and DNA. Through the reduction of oxidative stress, these antioxidants shield neural cells, thereby lowering the susceptibility to neurodegenerative conditions like Alzheimer's disease.

Anti-inflammatory Effects:

In addition to its antioxidant prowess, oregano's phenolic compounds also showcase anti-inflammatory properties. Chronic inflammation is a known factor in various health complications, including neurodegenerative disorders and chronic diseases. Through its anti-inflammatory actions, oregano aids in shielding neural cells and promoting overall brain health.

Neural Protection:

Oregano's antioxidant and anti-inflammatory properties work together to protect neural cells. This dual action helps prevent cognitive decline and supports brain function. Additionally, oregano's phenolic compounds may play a role in preventing neurodegenerative disorders by reducing oxidative stress and inflammation, key factors in the development of these conditions.

Medicinal Applications:

Beyond its neural protection, oregano has traditionally been used in folk medicine to alleviate various ailments, including asthma, bronchitis, and digestive issues. Its phytochemicals contribute to these benefits, making it a valuable herb for maintaining overall health.

3.5.6. Thyme and its Bioactive Profile

Thyme is a versatile herb native to the Mediterranean region, belonging to the Lamiaceae family. It has been recognized for centuries for its culinary, medicinal, and cosmetic uses. Thyme functions as an herb and antioxidant and plays a key role in protecting neural cells (Halat et al., 2022).

Nutritional and Chemical Composition:

Thyme is rich in nutrients, including vitamins, minerals, proteins, and fibers. Its chemical composition varies based on its geographical location, but it generally consists of antioxidants and flavonoids, which contribute to its therapeutic potential.

Therapeutic Properties:

Thyme's essential oils, particularly thymol and carvacrol, offer multiple pharmacological benefits. These include:

- Antioxidant: Thyme's antioxidants play a crucial role in neutralizing free radicals, which are unstable molecules capable of causing harm to cells, proteins, and DNA. Through the reduction of oxidative stress, these antioxidants aid in safeguarding neural cells, thereby thwarting cognitive decline and mitigating the risk of neurodegenerative disorders like Alzheimer's disease.
- Anti-inflammatory: Thyme is known for its anti-inflammatory effects, which are effective in reducing inflammation throughout the body, including the brain. Chronic inflammation plays a significant role in numerous health problems, particularly neurodegenerative

diseases. Through its inflammation-reducing properties, thyme helps to enhance overall brain health and functionality.

- Antimicrobial: Thyme's antiviral, antibacterial, and antifungal properties make it valuable in preventing infections and maintaining health. In addition, thyme's ability to disrupt microbial biofilms adds to its medicinal benefits, potentially supporting immune function.

Culinary and Nutraceutical Uses:

Thyme's pungent flavor and rich nutritional content make it a valuable culinary herb. Additionally, its therapeutic properties contribute to its use as a nutraceutical, offering health benefits beyond its culinary applications.

Cultural Significance:

Thyme has a long history in Mediterranean and Greek culture. Its name is derived from the Greek word "thymos", meaning courage or strength. Throughout history, thyme has been used as a medicinal plant, with its therapeutic properties documented in Dioscorides' work. Over time, thyme's use spread globally, solidifying its status as a valuable herb.

3.5.7. Sage: Protecting Neural Cells

Sage is a popular herb known for its culinary uses, but it also possesses significant medicinal properties. It's part of the mint family, and its botanical name is Salvia officinalis. Historically, sage has been used for a variety of ailments, and recent research has shed light on its potential role in neuroprotection (Bordoloi et al., 2024).

Antioxidant Properties:

Sage is packed with antioxidant compounds, such as flavonoids, phenolic acids, and rosmarinic acid. These antioxidants combat oxidative stress, a harmful process caused by an imbalance between free radicals and antioxidants in the body. Oxidative stress is known to contribute to cellular damage, particularly in neural cells.

Neuroprotective Role:

- Oxidative Stress Prevention: The antioxidants in sage help protect neural cells by neutralizing free radicals. This prevents damage to the cells' DNA, proteins, and lipids, which is crucial for maintaining neural function and preventing neurodegenerative diseases.

- Anti-inflammatory Effects: Sage has anti-inflammatory properties that can further aid neural health. Inflammation in the brain is linked to various neurological disorders, such as Alzheimer's and Parkinson's. By reducing inflammation, sage can potentially lower the risk of these conditions.
- Memory and Cognitive Function: Studies have suggested that sage may enhance memory and cognitive function. This effect is partly due to its antioxidant and anti-inflammatory properties, which protect neural cells and improve overall brain health. Additionally, some research indicates that sage might inhibit the enzyme acetylcholinesterase, which breaks down acetylcholine, a neurotransmitter essential for memory and cognition (Bordoloi et al., 2024).

Herbal Applications:

Sage can be consumed as a tea, supplement, or extract, offering an accessible way to incorporate its benefits into one's diet. Herbalists and naturopathic doctors often recommend sage for its neuroprotective and antioxidant properties, making it an integral part of holistic health regimens.

3.5.8. Ginkgo Biloba: A Guardian of Neural Cells

Ginkgo Biloba is a unique tree with a long history of medicinal use, particularly in traditional Chinese medicine. The leaves of this ancient tree are rich in compounds that offer significant health benefits, especially for neural health. Let's explore how Ginkgo Biloba serves as both an herb and an antioxidant, protecting neural cells in several ways.

Antioxidant Properties:

Ginkgo Biloba contains potent antioxidants such as flavonoids and terpenoids. These compounds help neutralize harmful free radicals, which can damage cells, including neurons. By reducing oxidative stress, Ginkgo Biloba protects the integrity of neural cells, contributing to better overall brain health.

Neuroprotective Role:
- Cognitive Enhancement: Ginkgo Biloba is recognized for its ability to boost memory and cognitive abilities. Research indicates that it can increase cerebral blood flow, providing the brain with essential oxygen and nutrients needed for optimal function. This enhanced circulation can lead to better mental sharpness and improved memory retention.

- Anti-inflammatory Benefits: Persistent inflammation within the brain is associated with several neurological conditions. The anti-inflammatory effects of Ginkgo Biloba can help mitigate this inflammation, potentially reducing the incidence of neurodegenerative diseases such as Alzheimer's and Parkinson's.
- Neurotransmitter Balance: Ginkgo Biloba is thought to influence the balance of neurotransmitters, chemicals that transmit signals between nerve cells. By regulating neurotransmitter levels, Ginkgo Biloba may improve communication between neural cells, leading to better cognitive performance and overall brain health.

Herbal Applications:

Ginkgo Biloba is available in various forms, including supplements, extracts, and teas. Its versatility makes it easy to incorporate into one's diet, allowing individuals to reap its neuroprotective benefits.

3.5.9. Milk Thistle

Milk Thistle (Silybum marianum), a flowering plant indigenous to the Mediterranean region, is renowned for its medicinal properties, particularly its seeds, which harbor a potent compound called silymarin. While often recognized for its liver health benefits, Milk Thistle also offers advantages for neural health owing to its antioxidant and anti-inflammatory attributes.

Antioxidant Properties:

Milk Thistle contains silymarin, a complex of flavonoids with strong antioxidant capabilities. These antioxidants help neutralize free radicals, preventing oxidative stress, which is a key factor in cellular damage, including that of neural cells. By reducing oxidative stress, Milk Thistle helps preserve the integrity and function of neurons.

Neuroprotective Role:

- Oxidative Stress Reduction: Silymarin's antioxidant properties play a pivotal role in diminishing oxidative stress on neural cells. This protective mechanism shields neurons from damage and degeneration, thereby diminishing the likelihood of neurodegenerative disorders like Alzheimer's and Parkinson's disease.
- Anti-inflammatory Effects: Milk Thistle has anti-inflammatory properties that further contribute to neural health. Chronic inflammation in the brain is associated with a range of

neurological disorders. By reducing inflammation, Milk Thistle can help prevent or mitigate these conditions, promoting overall brain health.

- Liver-Brain Connection: Milk Thistle's benefits for liver health indirectly support neural health. A healthy liver can process toxins more effectively, reducing the risk of harmful substances affecting the brain. This connection emphasizes the holistic nature of Milk Thistle's medicinal properties.

Herbal Applications:

Milk Thistle is available in various forms, including supplements and teas, making it easy to incorporate into one's daily routine. Herbalists and naturopaths often recommend Milk Thistle for its overall health benefits, including its neuroprotective properties.

3.5.10. Ashwagandha

Ashwagandha, also known as withania somnifera, is an ancient medicinal herb rooted in Ayurvedic tradition. Commonly referred to as Indian ginseng or winter cherry, Ashwagandha has been recognized for its adaptogenic properties, offering a range of health benefits, including its role as a potent antioxidant.

Antioxidant Properties:

Ashwagandha's antioxidant properties primarily stem from its bioactive compounds, particularly its withanolides, flavonoids, and phenolic acids. These compounds contribute to the herb's ability to neutralize free radicals and protect against oxidative stress, which is linked to various health concerns such as neurodegenerative diseases, cardiovascular issues, and premature aging.

Mechanisms of Action:

- Free Radical Neutralization: The bioactive compounds in Ashwagandha serve as effective scavengers, neutralizing damaging free radicals. These radicals are reactive molecules capable of harming cells and tissues. By countering these effects, Ashwagandha reduces oxidative stress, thereby preventing cellular damage and enhancing overall health.
- Enhancing Enzyme Function: Research has shown that Ashwagandha can boost the performance of critical antioxidant enzymes such as superoxide dismutase (SOD), catalase, and glutathione peroxidase. These enzymes play a crucial role in decomposing harmful reactive oxygen species (ROS) and reducing oxidative damage.

- Neuroprotection: Studies suggest that Ashwagandha may protect neurons from oxidative stress-induced damage. Its compounds help reduce lipid peroxidation, which can lead to neurodegenerative conditions. This neuroprotective effect makes Ashwagandha particularly valuable in supporting brain health.

Research Evidence:
- Clinical Studies: Research has demonstrated Ashwagandha's efficacy in reducing markers of oxidative stress (Smith, Lopresti & Fairchild, 2023). In one study, participants taking Ashwagandha showed significant increases in antioxidant enzyme levels, coupled with reduced oxidative damage markers.
- Animal Studies: Animal models have illustrated Ashwagandha's protective effects against oxidative stress-induced damage (Mikulska et al., 2023). For example, in studies on rodents, Ashwagandha supplementation was found to reduce lipid peroxidation in the liver and enhance antioxidant enzyme activity.

Applications in Health and Wellness:
- Stress Management: By reducing oxidative stress, Ashwagandha helps manage chronic stress, which can otherwise lead to systemic inflammation and related health issues.
- Neurodegenerative Conditions: Ashwagandha's neuroprotective properties may contribute to reducing the risk or slowing the progression of neurodegenerative diseases, including Alzheimer's and Parkinson's.
- Anti-Aging: The herb's antioxidant properties can combat premature aging by minimizing oxidative damage to cells, tissues, and organs, potentially improving longevity and skin health.

3.5.11. Mint (Mentha)

Mint is a popular aromatic herb used worldwide for its culinary and medicinal properties. This herb includes various species, such as peppermint and spearmint, which are recognized for their refreshing taste and potent health benefits, including antioxidant activity.

Antioxidant Properties:

Mint's antioxidant potential arises from its polyphenols, flavonoids, and essential oils, particularly menthol and menthone.

Mechanisms of Action:
- Free Radical Scavenging: Mint's polyphenols and flavonoids serve as scavengers, neutralizing free radicals responsible for oxidative stress and cellular harm.
- Enzyme Modulation: Mint has the capacity to boost the activity of crucial antioxidant enzymes such as superoxide dismutase (SOD), catalase, and glutathione peroxidase, facilitating the breakdown of reactive oxygen species (ROS).
- Anti-Inflammatory Effects: Mint's antioxidant attributes also lend to its anti-inflammatory effects, diminishing inflammation induced by oxidative stress.

Applications:
- Digestive Health: Mint's antioxidant properties can help reduce inflammation in the digestive tract, soothing symptoms of indigestion and irritable bowel syndrome.
- Cardiovascular Health: By reducing oxidative stress and inflammation, mint may help support cardiovascular health and reduce the risk of heart-related issues.
- Neuroprotection: Mint's compounds may protect neurons from oxidative stress-induced damage, potentially reducing the risk of neurodegenerative diseases.

3.5.12. Cilantro

Cilantro (Coriandrum sativum), also known as coriander, is a versatile herb used in culinary and medicinal practices. The leaves and seeds offer distinct flavors and health benefits, particularly its antioxidant properties.

Antioxidant Properties:
Cilantro's antioxidant activity is attributed to its polyphenols, flavonoids, and essential oils, including linalool and camphor.

Mechanisms of Action:
- Free Radical Scavenging: Cilantro's polyphenols and flavonoids act as scavengers, neutralizing free radicals and reducing oxidative stress.

- Chelating Heavy Metals: Cilantro's compounds can bind to heavy metals, reducing their oxidative effects and protecting against cellular damage. In other words, cilantro leaves can produce a chelating effect and help remove heavy metals from the body.
- Anti-Inflammatory Effects: Cilantro's antioxidant properties contribute to its anti-inflammatory effects, reducing inflammation linked to oxidative stress.

Applications:
- Detoxification: Cilantro's ability to chelate heavy metals makes it useful in detoxification protocols, reducing oxidative stress caused by metal toxicity.
- Cardiovascular Health: Cilantro's compounds may help reduce oxidative stress and inflammation in the cardiovascular system, supporting heart health.
- Anti-Aging: Cilantro's antioxidant properties may contribute to reducing premature aging by minimizing oxidative damage to cells and tissues.

3.5.13. Chamomile

Chamomile (Matricaria chamomilla) is a popular herb known for its soothing properties. It's commonly used in teas and herbal remedies, offering a range of health benefits, including antioxidant activity.

Antioxidant Properties:
Chamomile's antioxidant properties are primarily attributed to its flavonoids, polyphenols, and essential oils, including apigenin and chamazulene.

Mechanisms of Action:
- Free Radical Scavenging: Chamomile's flavonoids and polyphenols act as scavengers, neutralizing free radicals and protecting against oxidative stress.
- Anti-Inflammatory Effects: Chamomile's antioxidant compounds contribute to its anti-inflammatory effects, reducing inflammation associated with oxidative stress.
- Neuroprotection: Chamomile's compounds may protect neurons from oxidative damage, reducing the risk of neurodegenerative diseases.

Applications:

- Stress Relief: Chamomile's antioxidant and anti-inflammatory properties help reduce oxidative stress, promoting relaxation and alleviating stress-related symptoms.
- Sleep Aid: Chamomile's antioxidant properties may help promote restful sleep by reducing stress and inflammation, contributing to overall well-being.
- Skin Health: Chamomile's antioxidants may help reduce oxidative damage to the skin, potentially preventing premature aging and maintaining healthy skin.

3.6 Antioxidant-Packed Recipes

Remedies incorporating antioxidant-rich foods and beverages into your daily routine is an effective way to support overall well-being. In this collection of recipes for antioxidant remedies, we explore simple and delicious teas and infusions that can be easily prepared at home. These recipes blend powerful antioxidant herbs and ingredients to provide a variety of health benefits, from boosting cognitive health to enhancing metabolic function. Whether you're looking for a daily antioxidant boost or a specific remedy to support your well-being, these recipes offer practical and enjoyable solutions.

3.6.1. Teas and Infusions

(1) Green Tea and Lemon Balm Infusion for Daily Antioxidant Boost

Ingredients:

1 teaspoon of loose green tea leaves or 1 green tea bag

1 tablespoon of dried lemon balm leaves

1-2 teaspoons of honey or agave syrup (optional, for sweetness)

1 cup of hot water

Instructions:
- Place the green tea leaves or tea bag and dried lemon balm leaves into a teapot or heatproof infuser.
- Pour the hot water over the leaves, covering them completely.
- Let the mixture steep for 5-7 minutes, allowing the antioxidants from the tea and lemon balm to infuse into the water.

- Strain the mixture or remove the tea bag.
- Optionally, stir in honey or agave syrup to taste.
- Serve hot and enjoy this antioxidant-rich infusion for a daily health boost.

(2) Rosemary and Thyme Morning Tea for Cognitive Health

Ingredients:

1 teaspoon of dried rosemary leaves

1 teaspoon of dried thyme leaves

1 cup of hot water

1-2 teaspoons of honey or lemon juice (optional, for taste)

Instructions:

- Place the rosemary and thyme leaves into a teapot or heatproof infuser.
- Pour the hot water over the leaves, covering them fully.
- Allow the mixture to steep for 5-10 minutes, extracting the antioxidants and aromatic oils from the herbs.
- Strain the mixture or remove the infuser.
- Optionally, stir in honey or lemon juice for added flavor.
- Serve hot, enjoying the invigorating blend to kick-start your day.

3.6.2. Tinctures and Extracts

(1) Ginseng Root Tincture for Immune System Support

Ingredients:

1 cup of dried ginseng root (sliced or chopped)

2 cups of high-proof vodka or another neutral spirit

A sterilized glass jar with a lid

Instructions:

- Place the dried ginseng root into the sterilized glass jar.
- Pour the vodka over the root, ensuring it is fully covered.

- Close the jar securely and keep it in a cool, dark location.
- Shake the jar once daily for 4-6 weeks, allowing the ginseng's compounds to infuse into the alcohol.
- After 4-6 weeks, strain the mixture through a fine mesh or cheesecloth, transferring the tincture into a clean, sterilized bottle.
- Store the tincture in a cool, dark place.
- Usage: Take 10-15 drops of the tincture diluted in a small amount of water, up to twice daily, for immune system support.

(2) Turmeric Extract for Anti-Inflammatory Effects

Ingredients:

1 cup of fresh turmeric root (grated or sliced)

2 cups of high-proof vodka or another neutral spirit

A sterilized glass jar with a lid

Instructions:

- Place the grated or sliced turmeric root into the sterilized glass jar.
- Pour the vodka over the turmeric, ensuring it is fully covered.
- Close the jar securely and keep it in a cool, dark location.
- Shake the jar once daily for 4-6 weeks, allowing the turmeric's compounds to infuse into the alcohol.
- After 4-6 weeks, strain the mixture through a fine mesh or cheesecloth, transferring the tincture into a clean, sterilized bottle.
- Store the tincture in a cool, dark place.
- Usage: Take 10-15 drops internally by diluting the tincture in a small amount of water, up to twice daily, for anti-inflammatory support.

3.6.3. Topical Applications

Antioxidants not only play a vital role in maintaining internal health, but they also offer significant benefits for skin care. Topical applications of antioxidant-rich ingredients can protect the skin from free radical damage, reduce inflammation, and support repair processes. This helps prevent premature aging, maintains skin elasticity, and addresses minor skin concerns.

In this collection of topical applications, we explore two potent antioxidant remedies designed to nourish and protect the skin. From a revitalizing serum infused with green tea and rosehip oil to a healing salve made with turmeric and beeswax, these remedies offer practical solutions for everyday skincare needs.

(1) Antioxidant Skin Serum using Green Tea and Rosehip

Ingredients:

1 tablespoon of green tea extract (or 1 tablespoon of strong green tea infusion)

1 tablespoon of rosehip oil

1 teaspoon of vitamin E oil

5 drops of lavender essential oil (optional, for fragrance)

A small glass bottle with a dropper

Instructions:

- In a small mixing bowl, combine the green tea extract, rosehip oil, and vitamin E oil.
- Stir well to blend the ingredients thoroughly.
- Add the lavender essential oil, mixing again until evenly distributed.
- Carefully pour the mixture into the glass bottle, using a funnel if needed.
- Seal the bottle with a dropper cap, and store it in a cool, dark place.
- Usage: Apply a few drops of the serum onto clean skin, gently massaging it in using circular motions. For best results, use it daily as part of your skincare routine.

(2) Healing Salve with Turmeric and Beeswax for Skin Repair

Ingredients:

1 tablespoon of turmeric powder

1/4 cup of coconut oil

1/4 cup of beeswax pellets

1 teaspoon of lavender essential oil (optional, for fragrance)

A small glass jar with a lid

Instructions:

- In a heatproof bowl, melt the coconut oil and beeswax pellets together, either in a microwave or over a double boiler.
- Stir in the turmeric powder until fully blended, creating a uniform mixture.
- Add the lavender essential oil, mixing thoroughly.
- Pour the mixture into a small glass jar and let it cool and solidify.
- Seal the jar with a lid, and store it in a cool, dark location.
- Usage: Apply a small amount of the salve onto the affected area, gently massaging it in. Repeat as needed to support skin healing.

3.6.4. Recipes for Boosting Antioxidant Intake: Smoothies and Nutritional Boosts

Antioxidants used in food can interact in various ways, leading to synergistic, additive, or antagonistic effects. When naturally occurring antioxidants are combined, they can produce synergistic interactions, enhancing their effectiveness and making them especially suitable for application in food systems.

(1) Antioxidant Berry and Spinach Smoothie with a Hint of Ashwagandha

Ingredients:

1 cup of mixed berries (such as blueberries, strawberries, and raspberries)

1 cup of fresh spinach leaves

1/2 cup of plain Greek yogurt

1/2 cup of almond milk or other plant-based milk

1 teaspoon of ashwagandha powder

1 tablespoon of honey or agave syrup (optional, for sweetness)

Instructions:
- Place all ingredients into a blender.
- Blend until smooth, making sure all ingredients are fully incorporated.
- Pour into a glass and enjoy immediately for a nutrient-rich, antioxidant boost.

(2) Detoxifying Green Juice with Kale, Cilantro, and a Touch of Milk Thistle

Ingredients:

1 cup of kale leaves

1/2 cup of fresh cilantro leaves

1 teaspoon of milk thistle extract or 1 tablespoon of milk thistle seeds

1 apple, cored and sliced

1 lemon, juiced

1 cup of water

Instructions:

- *Place all ingredients into a blender or juicer.*
- *Blend or juice until smooth and consistent.*
- *Strain the mixture through a fine mesh if needed, then pour into a glass and enjoy immediately.*

3.6.5. Recipes for Boosting Immunity

(1) Immune-Boosting Green Smoothie

Ingredients:

1 cup of fresh baby spinach

1/2 cup of fresh parsley leaves

1 cup of pineapple chunks

1 banana, peeled

1/2 cup of coconut water

1 teaspoon of spirulina powder

Instructions:

- Place all ingredients into a blender.
- Blend until smooth, ensuring all ingredients are well incorporated.
- Pour into a glass and enjoy immediately for an immune-boosting treat.

(2) Turmeric-Ginger Immunity Shot

Ingredients:

1 inch of fresh turmeric root, grated (or 1 teaspoon of turmeric powder)

1 inch of fresh ginger root, grated

1/2 cup of warm water

1 tablespoon of lemon juice

1 tablespoon of honey or agave syrup

Instructions:

- In a small bowl, combine the grated turmeric and ginger.
- Add the warm water, lemon juice, and honey, stirring well to blend.
- Strain the mixture through a fine mesh into a shot glass.
- Drink immediately for an immunity boost.

(3) Garlic Lemon Chicken Soup

Ingredients:

1 tablespoon of olive oil

1 onion, chopped

4 cloves of garlic, minced

2 chicken breasts, cubed

4 cups of chicken broth

1 lemon, juiced

1 teaspoon of thyme

Salt and pepper to taste

Instructions:

- Heat the olive oil in a sizable pot over medium heat.
- Sauté the onion and garlic until they soften.
- Cook the chicken until it's no longer pink.
- Pour in the chicken broth, followed by the addition of lemon juice and thyme.
- Let it simmer for about 20 minutes to blend the flavors.
- Season with salt and pepper according to your taste preferences, and serve the dish piping hot.

(4) Citrus Immunity-Boosting Salad

Ingredients:

One orange, peeled and cut into segments

One grapefruit, peeled and cut into segments

Half a cup of pomegranate seeds

One cup of assorted greens (like spinach or arugula)

One tablespoon olive oil

One tablespoon apple cider vinegar

One teaspoon honey

Salt and pepper, adjusted according to taste

Instructions:

- Mix the orange segments, grapefruit segments, pomegranate seeds, and mixed greens together in a spacious bowl.
- In a smaller bowl, blend the olive oil, apple cider vinegar, honey, salt, and pepper by whisking them thoroughly.
- Pour the dressing over the salad and toss everything together to ensure an even coating.
- Serve immediately.

(5) Elderberry Syrup

Ingredients:

One cup dried elderberries

Three cups of water

One stick of cinnamon

One tablespoon of freshly grated ginger root

One cup of honey

Instructions:

- In a saucepan, combine the elderberries, water, cinnamon stick, and ginger root.
- Bring to a boil, then reduce heat and simmer for 30 minutes, allowing the mixture to reduce by half.
- Strain the mixture through a fine mesh or cheesecloth, discarding the solids.
- Stir in the honey until fully dissolved.

- Store the syrup in a sterilized bottle in the refrigerator.
- Usage: Take 1-2 tablespoons daily for immune support.

(6) Probiotic-Rich Yogurt Parfait

Ingredients:

One cup plain Greek yogurt

Half a cup of granola

Half a cup of assorted berries (like blueberries, strawberries, and raspberries)

One tablespoon chia seeds

One tablespoon honey

Preparation Method:

- Arrange the yogurt, granola, and berries in layers in a serving bowl or glass.
- Add a sprinkle of chia seeds on top.
- Finish with a drizzle of honey before serving.

(7) Green Tea Immunity Infusion

Ingredients:

1 teaspoon loose green tea leaves or 1 green tea bag

1 cup hot water

1 teaspoon lemon juice

1 teaspoon honey (if desired)

Instructions:

- Place the green tea leaves or bag into a cup.
- Pour the hot water over the tea, letting it steep for 5-7 minutes.
- Once steeped, remove the tea leaves or bag, then mix in the lemon juice and honey.
- Serve while hot and savor immediately

(8) Immune-Boosting Stir-Frying

Ingredients:

1 tablespoon of olive oil

1 onion, chopped

1 bell pepper, sliced

1 zucchini, sliced

1 cup of broccoli florets

1 cup of cooked chicken breast, cubed

1 tablespoon of soy sauce

1 teaspoon of ginger root, grated

Instructions:

- *In a large skillet or wok, heat the olive oil over medium heat.*
- *Add the onion, bell pepper, zucchini, and broccoli, stirring until they begin to soften.*
- *Add the cooked chicken, soy sauce, and ginger, cooking for a few minutes until heated through.*
- *Serve hot, either alone or over rice or noodles.*

EXTRA CONTENT

Uncover a treasure trove of extra content and additional resources waiting for you to explore and enjoy.

As a personal gift from the author, you will have access to exclusive bonuses such as:

- **Complete video lessons by Barbara O'Neill** (Healing the Gut, How to Fight Chronic Fatigue, How to Improve Your Mental Health, and more)
- **Herbal Topical Remedies**: Crafting Salves, Balms, Creams, and Ointments for Natural Healing

Scan the QR code or follow the link below to access everything:

https://www.boundlesspublishingpress.com/herbal-medicine-paperback-extra

CHAPTER 4: BLOOD SUGAR AND CARDIOVASCULAR SUPPORT

4.1 Understanding Blood Sugar Regulation

Blood sugar regulation involves intricate physiological processes aimed at maintaining blood glucose levels within a narrow range, vital for overall bodily function and well-being. Glucose serves as the primary energy source for cells, and its levels are carefully managed through hormonal mechanisms, primarily involving insulin and glucagon, both secreted by the pancreas.

Key elements of blood sugar regulation include:

Insulin: Produced by pancreatic beta cells, insulin facilitates the uptake of glucose from the bloodstream into cells, particularly in muscle and liver cells. It also promotes the conversion of glucose into glycogen, stored in the liver and muscles for future use.

Glucagon: Secreted by pancreatic alpha cells, glucagon opposes the actions of insulin. It prompts the liver to break down glycogen into glucose (glycogenolysis) and release it into the bloodstream, elevating blood sugar levels when they fall too low.

Diet and Lifestyle: Blood sugar levels are influenced by food intake, particularly carbohydrates, which are broken down into glucose. Regular exercise can increase insulin sensitivity, and managing stress and sleep patterns can also contribute to stable glucose levels.

4.2 Mechanisms of Blood Sugar Regulation: How Your Body Maintains Balance

The mechanisms of blood sugar regulation involve several critical processes: glucose uptake by cells for energy, the release of insulin to facilitate this uptake, the storage and release of glucose as glycogen in the liver and muscles, the role of other hormones in influencing glucose levels, the overall maintenance of homeostasis, and the impact of various pathologies that can disrupt these finely tuned systems.

Glucose Uptake: After consuming food, particularly carbohydrates, the digestive system breaks it down into simpler sugars, mainly glucose, which enters the bloodstream. This increases blood sugar levels, signaling the body to take regulatory action.

Insulin Release: When blood glucose levels rise, the pancreas responds by releasing insulin, a hormone produced by its beta cells. Insulin is pivotal in aiding the uptake of glucose into cells, especially those in muscle, liver, and fat tissues. By facilitating this process, insulin effectively reduces blood glucose levels by either converting glucose into energy or storing it as glycogen in the liver and muscles.

Glycogen Storage: Insulin also promotes glycogen synthesis, where excess glucose is converted into glycogen and stored primarily in the liver and muscles. This acts as a reserve that can be broken down and released back into the bloodstream when glucose levels drop.

Glucagon Release: When blood glucose levels fall below a certain threshold, such as during fasting or exercise, the pancreas releases glucagon, a hormone produced by its alpha cells. Glucagon signals the liver to break down glycogen into glucose (glycogenolysis) and release it into the bloodstream, raising blood sugar levels.

Role of other Hormones: In addition to insulin and glucagon, other hormones contribute to blood sugar regulation. Adrenaline and cortisol, released during stress or the fight-or-flight response, can increase blood glucose levels by promoting gluconeogenesis, the creation of glucose from non-carbohydrate sources.

Homeostasis: The balance between insulin and glucagon, along with contributions from other hormones, maintains blood glucose levels within a narrow range, ensuring the body's cells receive a steady supply of energy.

Pathologies: Dysregulation of these processes can lead to chronic conditions like diabetes. Type 1 diabetes results from an autoimmune destruction of beta cells, reducing insulin production. In type 2 diabetes, insulin resistance develops, impairing the body's ability to respond to insulin, leading to elevated blood glucose levels.

4.3 Herbs for Blood Sugar Management

Maintaining balanced blood sugar levels is essential for overall health and wellbeing, particularly for those managing diabetes or other metabolic conditions. While conventional medications and lifestyle modifications are often at the forefront of treatment, the use of herbal remedies has garnered significant attention for their potential role in blood sugar management. Let us examine the mechanisms behind these herbs, how they can complement traditional treatments, and considerations for incorporating them into a comprehensive approach to blood sugar management.

4.3.1 Cinnamon: Its role in Enhancing Insulin Sensitivity

Cinnamon, a popular spice derived from the bark of Cinnamomum trees, has long been recognized for its potential medicinal properties, particularly in the realm of blood sugar management. One of its key benefits is its ability to enhance insulin sensitivity, making it a valuable natural aid for those looking to manage their blood sugar levels. Here's how cinnamon contributes to improving insulin sensitivity:

Insulin Mimetic Properties: Studies have shown that cinnamon contains bioactive compounds, such as cinnamaldehyde, that have insulin-mimetic properties. These compounds can help mimic the effects of insulin, facilitating glucose uptake into cells and thereby reducing blood glucose levels.

Improved Cellular Signaling: Cinnamon has been found to enhance the insulin signaling pathway by increasing the phosphorylation of insulin receptor substrates. This improvement in signaling allows cells, particularly muscle and liver cells, to respond more effectively to insulin, promoting glucose uptake and utilization.

Reduced Insulin Resistance: By enhancing insulin sensitivity, cinnamon helps reduce insulin resistance, a key factor in type 2 diabetes. Reduced insulin resistance allows the body to use insulin more effectively, helping to regulate blood glucose levels more efficiently.

Antioxidant Effects: Cinnamon also contains potent antioxidants that can reduce oxidative stress, a factor that contributes to insulin resistance. By reducing oxidative stress, cinnamon helps protect insulin receptors and maintain proper function, further supporting blood sugar regulation.

Dietary Incorporation: The use of cinnamon as a dietary supplement or added to foods and beverages provides a convenient way to reap its potential benefits. While cinnamon should not replace conventional treatments, incorporating it into a balanced diet can complement other efforts to manage blood sugar

4.3.2 Fenugreek: Benefits in glucose tolerance and lowering blood sugar levels

Fenugreek (Trigonella foenum-graecum) is a widely-used herb in traditional medicine, with its significance increasingly recognized due to its potential benefits for blood sugar management and glucose tolerance enhancement. Here's a breakdown of how fenugreek aids in regulating blood sugar:

Enhancing Glucose Tolerance: Research indicates that fenugreek can boost glucose tolerance, aiding the body in maintaining stable blood sugar levels post-meal. This attribute is especially advantageous for those with insulin resistance or a predisposition to diabetes.

Rich in Soluble Fiber: The seeds of fenugreek contain abundant soluble fiber, which transforms into a gel-like substance in the gut. This fiber moderates carbohydrate absorption, allowing for a steady introduction of glucose into the bloodstream and averting abrupt blood sugar spikes.

Improving Insulin Sensitivity: Fenugreek is believed to increase insulin sensitivity, thereby enhancing the cellular response to insulin. This heightened sensitivity aids in the absorption of glucose into cells, thereby lowering overall blood glucose levels and aiding in the prevention of hyperglycemia.

Reducing Blood Sugar Levels: Regular intake of fenugreek is linked to decreased fasting blood sugar levels. The cumulative effect of enhanced glucose tolerance, slowed carbohydrate absorption, and improved insulin response helps in maintaining consistent blood sugar levels.

Bioactive Compounds: Fenugreek contains compounds such as 4-hydroxyisoleucine and trigonelline, which have been shown to support blood sugar regulation. 4-hydroxyisoleucine stimulates insulin secretion, while trigonelline has been associated with improved glucose metabolism.

Incorporation into Diet: Fenugreek can be incorporated into the diet in various forms, including seeds, powders, or extracts. It can be added to meals, brewed as a tea, or taken as a supplement, providing a convenient way to harness its benefits.

4.3.3 Hawthorn: Benefits for Heart Muscle Strength and Cholesterol Regulation

Hawthorn (Crataegus spp.) is a shrub native to Europe, Asia, and North America, known for its small red berries, fragrant flowers, and thorny branches. For centuries, it has been used in traditional medicine for its potential benefits in supporting heart health. Here's how hawthorn contributes to cardiovascular wellbeing:

Heart Muscle Strength: Hawthorn contains flavonoids and procyanidins, compounds that are believed to improve heart muscle function. These compounds enhance the contraction of the heart muscle, potentially increasing the force of each heartbeat and improving overall cardiac output. This can lead to better circulation and oxygen delivery throughout the body, benefiting overall cardiovascular health.

Vasodilation: Hawthorn has vasodilatory properties, which means it helps widen blood vessels. This reduction in vascular resistance can lower blood pressure, reducing the workload on the heart and further supporting heart muscle function.

Cholesterol Regulation: Research indicates that hawthorn may contribute to cholesterol level regulation. The antioxidant characteristics of hawthorn's flavonoids aid in diminishing the oxidation of LDL (low-density lipoprotein) cholesterol, a crucial element in atherosclerosis. This condition involves the accumulation of plaque in the arteries. By thwarting LDL oxidation, hawthorn supports the maintenance of healthier blood vessels and diminishes the likelihood of cardiovascular diseases.

Anti-inflammatory Effects: Hawthorn also exhibits anti-inflammatory properties, which can help reduce inflammation in blood vessels. This further supports cardiovascular health by maintaining smooth and unobstructed blood flow.

Dietary and Supplement Forms: Hawthorn is accessible in diverse forms such as teas, tinctures, and supplements, facilitating its integration into daily routines. Nonetheless, it's advisable to seek guidance from a healthcare provider prior to initiating hawthorn supplementation. This ensures compatibility with existing treatments and health conditions, optimizing safety and efficacy.

4.3.4 Garlic: Its Effectiveness in Reducing Blood Pressure and Cholesterol Levels

Garlic (Allium sativum) has been widely recognized for its culinary and medicinal benefits for centuries. Among its many health benefits, garlic's potential to support cardiovascular health, particularly in reducing blood pressure and cholesterol levels, has garnered significant attention. Here's how garlic contributes to heart health:

Blood Pressure Reduction: Garlic contains a compound called allicin, which has vasodilatory properties. This means it helps relax and widen blood vessels, reducing vascular resistance and allowing for smoother blood flow. This vasodilation can contribute to lower blood pressure, reducing the workload on the heart and decreasing the risk of cardiovascular events such as heart attack and stroke.

Cholesterol Reduction: Garlic has been found to positively influence cholesterol levels. Studies suggest that regular consumption of garlic can lower total cholesterol and LDL (low-density lipoprotein) cholesterol levels, which are key contributors to plaque buildup in the arteries and the development of atherosclerosis. By reducing LDL cholesterol levels, garlic helps support healthier blood vessels and overall cardiovascular health.

Antioxidant Properties: Garlic boasts a wealth of antioxidants that serve to shield the body against oxidative stress. This is pivotal as oxidative stress has the potential to harm blood vessels and induce the oxidation of LDL cholesterol, a contributing factor to atherosclerosis. By mitigating oxidative stress, garlic aids in the preservation of healthier blood vessels and promotes optimal cholesterol levels.

Anti-inflammatory Effects: Garlic also has anti-inflammatory properties, which can help reduce inflammation in the cardiovascular system. This further supports smooth blood flow and lowers the risk of cardiovascular issues.

Dietary Incorporation: Garlic can be incorporated into the diet in various ways, from fresh garlic cloves added to dishes to garlic supplements. It provides a convenient means of supporting cardiovascular health alongside a balanced diet and other lifestyle modifications.

4.3.5 Ginger: Anti-inflammatory effects and implications for heart health.

Ginger (Zingiber officinale) is a versatile spice and medicinal root widely used across cultures. Beyond its culinary applications, ginger has gained recognition for its anti-inflammatory properties and potential benefits for cardiovascular health. Here's how ginger contributes to heart health:

Anti-inflammatory Effects: Ginger harbors potent bioactive compounds like gingerol and shogaol, renowned for their anti-inflammatory attributes. These compounds function by hindering the production of pro-inflammatory molecules like prostaglandins and cytokines. By curbing inflammation within the body, ginger aids in alleviating inflammatory conditions that may contribute to cardiovascular issues.

Reducing Vascular Inflammation: Persistent inflammation in blood vessels can foster the onset of atherosclerosis, marked by plaque accumulation within the arteries. This buildup has the potential to narrow blood vessels, impeding blood circulation and elevating the likelihood of heart attacks and strokes. Leveraging ginger's anti-inflammatory attributes can mitigate vascular inflammation, thereby fostering the maintenance of healthier blood vessels and diminishing the risk of cardiovascular incidents.

Antioxidant Benefits: Ginger is rich in antioxidants that help protect the cardiovascular system from oxidative stress, which can damage blood vessels and contribute to the oxidation of LDL (low-density lipoprotein) cholesterol. Oxidized LDL is a key factor in the formation of atherosclerotic plaques. By reducing oxidative stress, ginger helps maintain healthier blood vessels and cholesterol levels, further supporting cardiovascular health.

Blood Pressure Regulation: Studies suggest that ginger may help regulate blood pressure by promoting vasodilation and smooth muscle relaxation. This reduces vascular resistance, allowing for smoother blood flow and reducing the workload on the heart.

Dietary Incorporation: Ginger can be incorporated into the diet in various forms, including fresh ginger root, powders, teas, and supplements. Adding ginger to meals and beverages provides a convenient way to harness its cardiovascular benefits.

4.3.6 Bitter Melon: Mechanisms that Help in Reducing Blood Sugar Levels

Bitter melon (Momordica charantia) is not a herb but a tropical vegetable with a distinctive, bumpy exterior and a bitter taste. It has been widely used in traditional medicine for its potential benefits in managing blood sugar levels. Here's how bitter melon contributes to reducing blood sugar levels:

Insulin-Mimetic Properties: Bitter melon contains compounds that have insulin-mimetic properties, particularly charantin and polypeptide-p, which can help to lower blood sugar levels. These compounds mimic the action of insulin by promoting glucose uptake into cells, reducing the amount of glucose in the bloodstream.

AMPK Activation: Bitter melon has been found to activate AMP-activated protein kinase (AMPK), an enzyme involved in cellular energy regulation. AMPK activation promotes glucose uptake into muscle cells and increases glucose metabolism, contributing to lower blood sugar levels.

Glycogen Synthesis: Bitter melon also supports glycogen synthesis, which involves converting glucose into glycogen for storage in the liver and muscles. This reduces the amount of glucose circulating in the bloodstream and helps to maintain balanced blood sugar levels.

Gluconeogenesis Inhibition: Bitter melon has been shown to inhibit gluconeogenesis, the process by which the liver produces glucose from non-carbohydrate sources. This helps to prevent an unnecessary increase in blood sugar levels, particularly during fasting periods.

Antioxidant Effects: Bitter melon is rich in antioxidants that help reduce oxidative stress, a factor that can contribute to insulin resistance. By reducing oxidative stress, bitter melon helps maintain proper insulin receptor function, further supporting blood sugar regulation.

Dietary Incorporation: Bitter melon can be consumed in various forms, including as a vegetable, juice, or supplement. Incorporating bitter melon into the diet can provide a natural means of supporting balanced blood sugar levels.

4.4 Herbal Remedies and Recipes for Blood Sugar Management

Following are some recipes that can provide practical and delicious ways to support healthy blood sugar levels.

(1) Cinnamon and Clove Tea for Blood Sugar Balance

Cinnamon and clove tea is a soothing, aromatic beverage that can help support balanced blood sugar levels. Both spices are known for their potential benefits in improving insulin sensitivity and reducing blood sugar. Here's a simple recipe to prepare this beneficial tea:

Ingredients:
1 cup of water
1 cinnamon stick or 1 teaspoon of ground cinnamon
2-3 whole cloves
1-2 teaspoons of honey or a natural sweetener (optional)

Instructions:
- Boil Water: In a small pot, bring 1 cup of water to a boil.

- Add Spices: Once the water is boiling, add the cinnamon stick or ground cinnamon and the cloves.
- Simmer: Reduce the heat to low and let the spices simmer for about 10 minutes, allowing the flavors to infuse.
- Strain: After simmering, remove the pot from heat and strain the tea into a cup, removing the cinnamon stick and cloves.
- Sweeten (Optional): If desired, add honey or a natural sweetener to taste, stirring until dissolved.
- Serve: Enjoy the tea hot, sipping it slowly for maximum benefit.

Additional Tips:
For an extra touch of flavor, consider adding a slice of fresh ginger or a squeeze of lemon juice during the simmering process.

(2) Fenugreek-Spiced Quinoa and Chickpea Salad
Fenugreek seed powder can be a versatile addition to your diet, offering potential benefits for blood sugar management. Here is a simple recipe for incorporating fenugreek seed powder into a nutritious and delicious dish:

Ingredients:
Two cups of either water or vegetable broth

One 15-ounce can of chickpeas, drained and rinsed

One teaspoon of fenugreek seed powder

One teaspoon of cumin powder

One teaspoon of paprika

Half a teaspoon of turmeric powder

One tablespoon of olive oil

One medium cucumber, cut into dice

One cup of cherry tomatoes, sliced in halves

Half of a red onion, minced

One-fourth cup of freshly chopped parsley

Juice from half a lemon

Salt and pepper, adjusted to taste

Instructions:

- Cook Quinoa: Rinse the quinoa thoroughly under cold water. In a medium-sized pot, bring 2 cups of water or vegetable broth to a boil. Add the quinoa, cover, and simmer for about 15 minutes or until the water is absorbed. Fluff with a fork and set aside to cool.
- Mix Spices: In a small bowl, combine the fenugreek seed powder, cumin powder, paprika, turmeric powder, salt, and pepper.
- Prepare Chickpeas: In a large mixing bowl, combine the chickpeas with the spice mix, tossing until evenly coated.
- Assemble the Salad: Add the cooled quinoa to the chickpeas, followed by the diced cucumber, cherry tomatoes, red onion, and parsley. Drizzle the olive oil and lemon juice over the top and toss everything together until well mixed.
- Serve: Transfer the salad to serving dishes and enjoy it warm or cold.

Additional Tips:

- *Meal Prep*: This salad can be prepared in advance and stored in the refrigerator for up to 3 days, making it a convenient option for busy schedules.
- *Variations*: Feel free to customize the recipe by adding other ingredients such as olives, avocado, or other herbs like mint or cilantro.
- *Complementary Foods*: This dish pairs well with a variety of proteins, such as grilled chicken or tofu, or can be enjoyed as a complete vegetarian meal.

4.5 Herbal Remedies and Recipes for Cardiovascular Health

(1) Hawthorn Berry Tincture for Daily Heart Support

Hawthorn berry tincture is an effective way to support heart health regularly. The tincture is made by extracting the beneficial compounds of the hawthorn berries into alcohol, making it easy to consume in small doses. Here's how to prepare a hawthorn berry tincture:

Ingredients:

1 cup dried hawthorn berries

2 cups high-proof alcohol (such as vodka, at least 40% ABV)

1 clean, glass jar with a tight-fitting lid (16 oz or larger)

Cheesecloth or fine mesh strainer

Small dark glass dropper bottles for storage

Instructions:
- Prepare the Jar: Place the dried hawthorn berries into the glass jar.
- Add Alcohol: Pour the alcohol over the berries, ensuring they are fully submerged. The alcohol acts as a solvent, extracting the beneficial compounds from the berries.
- Seal and Steep: Secure the lid tightly on the jar and give it a good shake. Place the jar in a cool, dark place for at least 4 weeks. Shake it occasionally. This allows time for the active compounds to infuse into the alcohol.
- Strain the Mixture: After 4 weeks, strain the mixture through a cheesecloth or fine mesh strainer into a clean bowl or container. This procedure helps separate the liquid tincture from the berries.
- Bottle the Tincture: Pour the strained tincture into dark glass dropper bottles for storage. Dark glass helps protect the tincture from light, preserving its potency.
- Dosage: For daily heart support, take 1-2 droppers of the tincture (approximately 1-2 ml) under the tongue or mixed into a glass of water or juice. Consult a healthcare professional for specific dosage recommendations.

Additional Tips:
- *Shelf Life*: Properly stored in a dark, cool place, the tincture can last up to a year or more.
- *Customizing*: The tincture can be customized by adding other heart-supportive herbs, such as motherwort or lemon balm, to the mixture during the steeping process.

(2) Garlic and Lemon Tonic for Maintaining Healthy Arteries

Garlic and lemon tonic is a refreshing and health-boosting drink that supports cardiovascular health by helping to maintain healthy arteries. This tonic combines the benefits of garlic's cholesterol-lowering and blood-pressure-regulating properties with lemon's antioxidants and vitamin C. Here's how to prepare this simple yet effective tonic:

Ingredients:

1 head of garlic

2 cups of water

Juice of 2 lemons

1 tablespoon honey (optional)

Instructions:

- Prepare Garlic: Peel the garlic cloves and finely chop or crush them to release the beneficial compounds. Alternatively, you can use a garlic press.
- Boil Water: In a small pot, bring 2 cups of water to a boil.
- Add Garlic: Once the water is boiling, add the chopped or crushed garlic. Reduce the heat and let it simmer for about 5 minutes, allowing the beneficial compounds to infuse into the water.
- Remove from Heat: After simmering, remove the pot from heat and let it cool slightly.
- Strain: Strain the mixture into a clean container or jug, removing the garlic solids.
- Add Lemon Juice: Stir in the juice of 2 lemons. The acidity of the lemon juice complements the garlic's flavor and provides additional health benefits.
- Sweeten (Optional): If desired, add 1 tablespoon of honey or a natural sweetener to taste, stirring until dissolved.
- Serve: Transfer the tonic into a glass and enjoy. This tonic can be consumed warm or cold.

Additional Tips:

- *Storage*: The tonic can be stored in a refrigerator for up to 3 days, making it convenient for regular consumption.
- *Customizing*: To further enhance the tonic, consider adding a slice of fresh ginger or a dash of cayenne pepper, which also offer cardiovascular benefits

CHAPTER 5: DETOX AND DIGESTIVE WELLNESS

5.1 Understanding Detoxification

5.1.1. The role of detoxification in overall health

Detoxification plays a crucial role in overall health by helping the body remove toxins and harmful substances, which can accumulate over time due to environmental pollutants, unhealthy diets, and stress. This natural process is primarily handled by the liver, kidneys, and digestive system, which work together to filter and eliminate waste products.

5.1.2. Key Roles of the Liver, Kidneys, and Skin in the Body's Detoxification System

The liver and kidneys are crucial organs in the body's detoxification processes. They work in tandem to filter and eliminate toxins, waste products, and other harmful substances from the body, maintaining overall health and homeostasis. Regular detoxification supports various aspects of overall health, including improved energy levels, better mental clarity, weight management, and reduced risk of chronic diseases. It also supports immune function, making the body more resilient to illnesses. Here's how each organ contributes:

Liver Function:
- *Metabolizing Toxins*: The liver is the primary organ for metabolizing toxins. It processes substances such as drugs, alcohol, and chemicals, converting them into less harmful compounds. The liver's enzymes, particularly the cytochrome P450 family, play a key role in breaking down these toxins.
- *Conjugation*: After metabolizing toxins, the liver often conjugates them with molecules like glucuronic acid, making them water-soluble. This allows the toxins to be excreted more easily through the kidneys or digestive system.
- *Bile Production*: The liver produces bile, which aids in the digestion and absorption of fats. Bile also helps to eliminate fat-soluble toxins and cholesterol from the body by carrying them into the digestive tract, where they can be excreted.
- *Storage*: The liver stores essential nutrients, such as vitamins and minerals, which are crucial for maintaining health and supporting the body's ability to manage toxins and stress.

Kidney Function:

- *Filtering the Blood*: The kidneys act as filters for the blood, removing waste products, toxins, and excess substances. Blood flows through the kidneys, where it is filtered, allowing toxins and waste products to be excreted in urine.
- *Excretion*: The kidneys excrete various waste products, including urea, creatinine, and drugs, through urine. This prevents the buildup of harmful substances in the body.
- *Electrolyte Balance*: The kidneys maintain a proper balance of electrolytes, such as sodium and potassium, which is essential for normal cellular functions. They also help regulate the body's pH balance by adjusting the excretion of acids and bases.
- *Fluid Balance*: The kidneys play a key role in regulating fluid balance by controlling the amount of water reabsorbed or excreted in urine. This helps maintain blood pressure and supports the body's overall detoxification capacity.

The Skin:

The skin contributes to the body's detoxification processes in several ways:
- *Excretion of Toxins*: The skin helps to excrete toxins and waste products through sweat. Sweat glands release perspiration, which contains various waste materials such as urea, salts, and ammonia. This helps reduce the overall toxic load in the body, complementing the liver and kidneys in their detoxification roles.
- *Barrier Function*: The skin acts as a protective barrier, preventing harmful substances and microorganisms from entering the body. By shielding the internal organs from environmental toxins, allergens, and pathogens, the skin reduces the potential for systemic toxicity.
- *Sebum Production*: The sebaceous glands in the skin secrete sebum, an oily substance that lubricates and protects the skin. Sebum also contains antimicrobial properties, which help prevent infection and reduce the risk of toxins entering the body through cuts or wounds.
- *Temperature Regulation*: The skin's ability to regulate body temperature through sweating helps prevent overheating, which could otherwise impair bodily functions, including those involved in detoxification.
- *Microbiome Balance*: The skin hosts a diverse microbiome of bacteria, fungi, and other microorganisms. A balanced microbiome helps protect against harmful pathogens, reducing the risk of infections that can strain the body's detoxification systems.

5.2 Key Herbs and Their Detoxifying Properties

5.2.1 Milk Thistle: Silymarin as a Liver Protector and Regenerator

Milk thistle, scientifically known as Silybum marianum, is a plant that has been used for centuries for its medicinal properties, particularly in supporting liver health. The key active compound in milk thistle is silymarin, a complex of flavonolignans, which has been shown to have potent liver-protective and regenerative properties. Here's how silymarin supports liver health:

- *Antioxidant Properties*: Silymarin acts as a powerful antioxidant, neutralizing free radicals and reducing oxidative stress in the liver. This helps to protect liver cells from damage caused by toxins, alcohol, and other harmful substances, preventing the onset of liver diseases such as cirrhosis and fatty liver disease.
- *Anti-inflammatory Effects*: Silymarin exhibits anti-inflammatory properties by inhibiting the release of pro-inflammatory cytokines. This reduces inflammation in the liver, helping to prevent chronic conditions such as hepatitis and non-alcoholic fatty liver disease (NAFLD).
- *Liver Cell Regeneration*: Silymarin stimulates the regeneration of hepatocytes, the main cells of the liver. This regenerative capacity is crucial for recovering from liver damage caused by alcohol, drugs, or other toxins. By promoting new cell growth, silymarin helps restore liver function and improves overall liver health.
- *Inhibition of Toxin Binding*: Silymarin prevents toxins from binding to liver cells by altering the structure of cell membranes. This helps reduce toxin uptake and accumulation in the liver, protecting it from damage caused by harmful substances.
- *Improving Liver Function*: Studies have shown that milk thistle can improve liver function tests in people with liver disorders. This includes reduced levels of liver enzymes such as ALT and AST, which are markers of liver damage.
- *Protection Against Alcohol-Induced Liver Damage*: Silymarin has been shown to mitigate liver damage caused by excessive alcohol consumption. It inhibits lipid peroxidation and reduces inflammation, minimizing alcohol-induced damage and supporting recovery.

5.2.2. Dandelion Root and Leaf: Benefits for Liver and Kidney Detox

Dandelion (Taraxacum officinale) is a flowering plant known for its medicinal properties, particularly its benefits for liver and kidney health. Both the root and leaves of the dandelion have been used traditionally to support detoxification, and contemporary research continues to validate their efficacy (Fan et al., 2023). Dandelion root and leaves play a key role in the detoxification of the liver and kidneys:

Dandelion Root for Liver Health

- *Liver Stimulant*: Dandelion root acts as a liver tonic, stimulating bile production. This increase in bile helps in the digestion and absorption of fats, while also aiding in the elimination of toxins and waste products through the digestive tract.

- *Anti-inflammatory Properties*: The root has anti-inflammatory properties that help reduce inflammation in the liver, which can contribute to various liver conditions such as hepatitis and non-alcoholic fatty liver disease (NAFLD). This anti-inflammatory effect helps support overall liver health and function.

- *Antioxidant Benefits*: Dandelion root contains antioxidants, including flavonoids and phenolic compounds, which help neutralize free radicals and reduce oxidative stress in the liver. This protective effect helps prevent liver damage caused by toxins and environmental pollutants.

Dandelion Leaves for Kidney Health

- *Diuretic Properties*: Dandelion leaves act as a natural diuretic, increasing urine output and supporting the kidneys in filtering and eliminating waste products and toxins. This diuretic effect helps reduce the burden on the kidneys, preventing toxin buildup and supporting overall kidney health.

- *Electrolyte Balance*: Unlike synthetic diuretics that can lead to potassium depletion, dandelion leaves are rich in potassium, helping to maintain electrolyte balance even as they increase urine output. This helps support kidney function without causing an imbalance in essential minerals.

- *Detoxification Support*: The diuretic and electrolyte-balancing properties of dandelion leaves contribute to overall detoxification. By promoting the excretion of waste products and preventing toxin accumulation, dandelion leaves help maintain kidney health and reduce the risk of kidney-related conditions.

- *Nutritional Benefits*: Both dandelion root and leaves are rich in vitamins and minerals, including vitamins A, C, and K, as well as iron and calcium. These nutrients support overall health and play a role in maintaining the function of the liver, kidneys, and other organs involved in detoxification.

5.2.3. Burdock Root: Its Role in Purifying Blood and Promoting Skin Health

Burdock root (Arctium lappa) has been used for centuries in traditional medicine for its medicinal properties, particularly its ability to purify the blood and promote skin health. Here's how burdock root plays a crucial role in these areas:

Blood Purification

-   *Diuretic Properties*: Burdock root acts as a natural diuretic, promoting increased urine output. This helps remove waste products, toxins, and excess fluids from the blood, supporting the body's detoxification processes.
-   *Lymphatic System Support*: Burdock root helps stimulate the lymphatic system, which plays a key role in filtering and removing waste products from the blood. By supporting lymphatic function, burdock root aids in the overall detoxification process and helps prevent toxin buildup.
-   *Antioxidant Properties*: Burdock root contains antioxidants such as quercetin and luteolin, which neutralize free radicals and reduce oxidative stress in the blood. This helps prevent damage to blood cells and supports overall blood health.
-   *Liver Support*: Burdock root can also aid liver function, which contributes to blood purification. By supporting liver health, burdock root helps the liver metabolize toxins and waste products more efficiently, contributing to cleaner blood.

Skin Health

-   *Antibacterial and Anti-inflammatory Properties*: Burdock root has antibacterial and anti-inflammatory properties, which can help reduce skin inflammation and prevent bacterial infections. This makes it useful in treating skin conditions such as acne, eczema, and psoriasis.
-   *Detoxification and Skin Clarity*: By supporting overall detoxification and blood purification, burdock root can help improve skin clarity. Toxin buildup and blood impurities can contribute to skin issues such as blemishes and breakouts, and burdock root's detoxifying effects help reduce these issues, leading to clearer, healthier skin.

Nutritional Benefits

Burdock root contains essential vitamins and minerals, including vitamins A, C, and E, which are important for skin health. These nutrients support collagen production, improve skin elasticity, and promote overall skin repair and regeneration.

Digestive Support

Burdock root is a source of inulin, a prebiotic fiber that supports gut health by promoting the growth of beneficial bacteria. A healthy gut microbiome contributes to overall health, including skin health, by reducing inflammation and improving nutrient absorption.

5.3 Herbal Remedies and Recipes for Detoxification

(a) Milk Thistle Seed Decoction for Liver Support

Ingredients:

1 tablespoon of crushed milk thistle seeds

3 cups of water

Instructions:

- Crush the Seeds: Start by crushing the milk thistle seeds using a mortar and pestle or a spice grinder. This helps to release the active compounds, silymarin, making them more available during the brewing process.
- Boil Water: Bring 3 cups of water to a boil in a small saucepan.
- Add the Milk Thistle Seeds: Once the water is boiling, add the crushed milk thistle seeds to the saucepan.
- Simmer: Reduce the heat and let the mixture simmer gently for 20 minutes. This slow cooking process helps extract the silymarin from the seeds into the water.
- Strain: After simmering, remove the saucepan from the heat. Strain the decoction through a fine mesh sieve or a piece of cheesecloth into a clean container. Press or squeeze the seed residue to extract as much liquid as possible.
- Serve: The milk thistle seed decoction can be consumed warm or cooled. It has a slightly bitter flavor, which you can soften with a little honey or lemon if desired.
- Dosage/Frequency: Drink 1 cup of the decoction 1 to 2 times daily. This regimen can be particularly beneficial for those looking to support liver health due to exposure to toxins, a history of liver issues, or as a preventive measure.

(b) Dandelion and Burdock Root Tea for Comprehensive Detox

Ingredients:

1 tablespoon dried dandelion root

1 tablespoon dried burdock root

4 cups of water

Optional: Honey, lemon, or other natural sweeteners for taste

Instructions:

- Prepare the Roots: Begin by crushing or breaking up the dried dandelion and burdock roots to help release their active compounds. You can use a mortar and pestle or simply chop them finely with a knife.
- Boil the Water: In a medium-sized saucepan, bring 4 cups of water to a boil.
- Add the Roots: Once the water is boiling, add the prepared dandelion and burdock roots to the saucepan.
- Simmer: Reduce the heat and let the mixture simmer for 10–15 minutes. This allows the active compounds in the roots to infuse into the water.
- Strain: After simmering, remove the saucepan from heat and strain the mixture through a fine mesh sieve or cheesecloth into a teapot or heat-resistant pitcher. This removes the solid pieces, leaving a clear, detoxifying tea.
- Serve: Pour the tea into cups and enjoy. If desired, add honey, lemon, or other natural sweeteners to taste.

5.4 Herbal Remedies for Digestive Wellness

5.4.1 Peppermint: Easing Digestive Spasms and Discomfort

Peppermint (Mentha piperita) has been widely used in traditional and modern medicine for its medicinal properties, particularly its ability to ease digestive spasms and discomfort. The active compounds in peppermint, especially menthol, contribute to its soothing effects on the digestive system. Peppermint can help alleviate digestive issues in many ways:

- *Antispasmodic Properties*: Peppermint's primary active compound, menthol, acts as an antispasmodic, relaxing the smooth muscles of the digestive tract. This helps alleviate spasms in the intestines, which are often associated with conditions such as irritable bowel syndrome (IBS) and functional dyspepsia.

- *Reducing Bloating and Gas*: Peppermint's relaxing effect on the digestive tract helps reduce bloating and gas by promoting the passage of gas through the intestines. This helps relieve discomfort and pressure, contributing to overall digestive well-being.
- *Improving Digestion*: Peppermint aids digestion by stimulating the flow of digestive juices, including bile. This helps break down fats and improves nutrient absorption, reducing symptoms of indigestion and promoting overall digestive health.
- *Anti-inflammatory Properties*: Peppermint has anti-inflammatory properties that can help soothe inflammation in the digestive tract, reducing discomfort associated with conditions such as gastritis and colitis.
- *Cooling Effect*: Menthol, found in peppermint, has a cooling effect that can help soothe irritated digestive tissues. This provides immediate relief from discomfort, especially in cases of heartburn or acid reflux.

Forms of Consumption
- *Peppermint Tea:* One popular and effective way to use peppermint for digestive relief is by drinking peppermint tea. Steeping peppermint leaves in hot water releases its active compounds, providing a soothing beverage that helps alleviate digestive issues.
- *Peppermint Oil:* Peppermint oil capsules are another option for easing digestive discomfort. These capsules deliver a concentrated dose of menthol directly to the digestive tract, providing targeted relief from spasms and discomfort.

(a) Ginger: Stimulating Digestion and Reducing Nausea

Ginger supports digestive health in many ways.

- *Digestive Stimulant*: Ginger has compounds like gingerols and shogaols, which stimulate the digestive system by enhancing the production of digestive enzymes and bile. This aids in the breakdown and absorption of nutrients from food, improving overall digestion and reducing symptoms of indigestion.
- *Antiemetic Properties*: Ginger is well-known for its antiemetic (anti-nausea) properties. It can help alleviate nausea caused by motion sickness, pregnancy, or medical treatments such as chemotherapy. The precise mechanism by which ginger reduces nausea is still being studied,

but it is believed to involve interactions with serotonin receptors in the gut, which helps regulate gastric motility.

- *Reducing Bloating and Gas*: Ginger's carminative properties help reduce bloating and gas by relaxing the smooth muscles of the digestive tract. This promotes the passage of gas, reducing discomfort and distension.
- *Anti-inflammatory Effects*: Ginger has anti-inflammatory properties that help soothe inflammation in the digestive tract. This can reduce discomfort associated with conditions such as gastritis or inflammatory bowel disease, supporting overall digestive health.
- *Antioxidant Benefits*: Ginger contains antioxidants that help neutralize free radicals and reduce oxidative stress in the digestive system. This helps protect the digestive tract from damage caused by toxins and environmental pollutants.

Forms of Consumption

- *Ginger Tea*: One of the simplest ways to incorporate ginger into your routine is by making ginger tea. This is prepared by steeping freshly sliced or grated ginger root in hot water for 10–15 minutes. The resulting tea can be consumed warm or cooled, providing immediate digestive relief.
- *Ginger Supplements*: Ginger supplements, available in capsules or tablet form, offer a concentrated dose of ginger's active compounds. They are convenient for targeted relief from nausea or digestive discomfort.
- *Culinary Uses*: Incorporating ginger into cooking provides a flavorful way to support digestive health. Grated ginger can be added to stir-fries, soups, or smoothies, providing both flavor and digestive benefits

5.4.2 Fennel: Benefits for Gas and Bloating Relief

Fennel (Foeniculum vulgare) is a flavorful herb that has been used for centuries for its medicinal properties, particularly in supporting digestive health. Its ability to relieve gas and bloating makes it a valuable natural remedy for digestive discomfort. Fennel contributes to alleviating these issues due to its carminative and anti-inflammatory properties, as well as by acting as a digestive stimulant.

- *Carminative Properties:* Fennel contains volatile oils such as anethole, fenchone, and estragole, which give it carminative properties. These compounds help relax the smooth muscles of the digestive tract, allowing gas to pass more easily. This reduces bloating and relieves discomfort associated with trapped gas.

- *Antispasmodic Effects*: The compounds in fennel also have antispasmodic effects, reducing spasms in the digestive tract that can contribute to gas buildup and bloating. This makes fennel an effective remedy for digestive issues such as irritable bowel syndrome (IBS) and functional dyspepsia.

- *Digestive Stimulant*: Fennel stimulates the secretion of digestive enzymes, aiding in the breakdown of food and absorption of nutrients. This helps prevent indigestion, which can lead to bloating and gas, and promotes overall digestive health.

- *Anti-inflammatory Properties*: Fennel has anti-inflammatory properties that can help soothe inflammation in the digestive tract. This reduces discomfort associated with conditions such as gastritis and colitis, contributing to a healthier digestive system.

- *Antioxidant Benefits:* Fennel is rich in antioxidants, including flavonoids and phenolic compounds, which help neutralize free radicals and reduce oxidative stress in the digestive system. This protects the digestive tract from damage caused by toxins and environmental pollutants.

Forms of Consumption

- *Fennel Tea*: One of the simplest ways to incorporate fennel into your routine is by drinking fennel tea. This is prepared by steeping 1–2 teaspoons of crushed fennel seeds or a handful of fresh fennel leaves in a cup of hot water for 10 minutes. The resulting tea can be consumed warm or cooled, providing immediate relief from gas and bloating.

- *Fennel Seeds*: Chewing fennel seeds after a meal can also aid digestion and reduce gas buildup. The volatile oils in the seeds help relax the digestive tract and promote the passage of gas.

- *Culinary Uses*: Fennel can be incorporated into meals in various forms, including fresh fennel bulbs, leaves, or seeds. This provides both flavor and digestive benefits, helping to prevent bloating and gas.

5.5 Recipes for Digestive Health

(a) Peppermint Tea

Instructions:

- Steep 1–2 teaspoons of dried peppermint leaves or a handful of fresh leaves in a cup of hot water for 5–10 minutes.
- Strain the leaves and enjoy the tea warm or cooled.

(b) Peppermint and Ginger Digestive Tincture

This tincture combines the digestive benefits of peppermint and ginger, making it a convenient and potent remedy for digestive discomfort.

Ingredients:

1/4 cup dried peppermint leaves

1/4 cup freshly grated ginger root (or 2 tablespoons dried ginger root)

1 cup vodka or brandy (high-proof alcohol, 40% or higher)

A glass jar with a tight-fitting lid

A dropper bottle for storing the tincture

Instructions:

- Prepare the Jar: Place the dried peppermint leaves and ginger root into the glass jar.
- Add the Alcohol: Pour the vodka or brandy over the herbs, ensuring they are fully submerged.
- Seal and Shake: Seal the jar tightly and shake it thoroughly to mix the ingredients.
- Infuse: Place the jar in a cool, dark place for 4–6 weeks, shaking it occasionally. This allows the active compounds from the peppermint and ginger to infuse into the alcohol.
- Strain: After 4–6 weeks, strain the mixture through a fine mesh sieve or cheesecloth into a clean container.
- Store: Transfer the strained tincture into a dropper bottle for easy use.
- Usage: Take 10–20 drops of the tincture in a small amount of water or directly on the tongue, as needed, to relieve digestive discomfort such as indigestion, bloating, or nausea.

(c) Fennel Seed Infusion for After-Meal Digestive Comfort:

This fennel seed infusion provides a simple and soothing remedy for digestive discomfort after meals.

Ingredients:

1 teaspoon fennel seeds

1 cup hot water

Instructions:

- Crush the Seeds: Crush the fennel seeds lightly with a mortar and pestle or the back of a spoon to release their oils.
- Steep: Place the crushed fennel seeds in a cup and pour hot water over them. Allow the infusion to steep for 10 minutes.
- Strain: After steeping, strain the infusion through a fine mesh sieve into another cup, removing the seeds.
- Serve: Drink the fennel seed infusion warm after meals to promote digestive comfort.

CHAPTER 6: MOOD, STRESS MANAGEMENT AND IMPROVED SLEEP

This chapter focuses on the antidepressant properties, stress resilience enhancement, anxiety alleviation, and relaxation promotion of key herbs and their associated benefits.

6.1 Herbs for Stress and Anxiety

(a) Ashwagandha and its role in Enhancing Resilience to Stress

Ashwagandha is an adaptogenic herb renowned for its stress-relieving properties. It helps to lower cortisol levels, which is often referred to as the "stress hormone" (National Institutes of Health, 2023). Following are the key benefits of Ashwagandha in reducing stress and anxiety:

- Cortisol Reduction: Ashwagandha has been shown in studies to reduce cortisol levels significantly, which can help alleviate the physical effects of stress. By balancing cortisol, the herb can also reduce other stress-related symptoms, including weight gain and hormonal imbalances.
- Improved Resilience: The herb enhances the body's resilience to stress, allowing individuals to manage stressors more effectively. This makes it useful for those facing chronic or high levels of stress.
- Calming Effect: Ashwagandha has been linked to a reduction in anxiety symptoms. Its calming effect on the nervous system can help individuals feel more relaxed and grounded.
- Mood Improvement: Regular use of Ashwagandha has been associated with improved mood and a decrease in feelings of anxiety and depression. This makes it valuable not only for stress management but also for overall mental health.

(b) St. John's Wort and its Antidepressant Properties

St. John's Wort is a popular herbal remedy recognized for its antidepressant properties and its potential to alleviate stress and anxiety. The key benefits of St. John's Wort: are

- *Mood Enhancement*: St. John's Wort is believed to increase levels of neurotransmitters like serotonin, dopamine, and norepinephrine, which can improve mood and help alleviate symptoms of depression. This has made it a popular natural alternative to traditional antidepressants.

- *Anxiety Reduction*: The herb's ability to balance neurotransmitter levels can also help reduce anxiety symptoms, offering a calming effect. This makes it particularly useful for those experiencing stress and anxiety alongside depressive symptoms.
- *Stress Management*: St. John's Wort may help to manage stress by stabilizing mood and promoting a more positive outlook. This can help individuals better cope with everyday stressors and challenges.
- *Insomnia Relief*: For those experiencing stress and anxiety-related insomnia, St. John's Wort has been reported to help improve sleep quality. Better sleep can contribute to reduced stress and a healthier overall mental state.

(c) Lavender and its Calming and Sedative Effects

Lavender is a versatile herb known for its calming and sedative properties, making it a valuable tool for managing stress and anxiety. Following are the key benefits of lavender:

- *Calming Effect*: Lavender has been used for centuries for its relaxing aroma, which can help reduce stress and promote a sense of calm. The scent alone has been shown to lower blood pressure and heart rate, helping to create a tranquil environment.
- *Anxiety Reduction*: Lavender's calming properties extend beyond its aroma. Consuming lavender, whether through teas, capsules, or essential oils, has been linked to reduced anxiety levels. Its soothing effects can help mitigate feelings of tension and unease.
- *Improved Sleep*: Lavender is often used to promote restful sleep, which is essential for stress management. The herb's calming effects can help individuals fall asleep faster and stay asleep longer, reducing stress-related insomnia.
- *Mood Stabilization*: Lavender's impact on the nervous system can contribute to a more balanced mood. This is particularly helpful for those experiencing mood swings or irritability related to stress and anxiety.

(d) Chamomile and its ability to Ease Anxiety and Promote Relaxation

Chamomile is a widely used herb, renowned for its ability to ease anxiety and promote relaxation. The key benefits of chamomile are:

- *Anxiety Reduction*: Chamomile has been traditionally used for its calming properties, making it an effective natural remedy for anxiety. Drinking chamomile tea or using chamomile supplements can help alleviate feelings of tension and stress.
- *Relaxation*: Chamomile's soothing effect on the nervous system helps to promote relaxation, making it a valuable tool for those experiencing stress. This relaxation can help balance emotions, reduce irritability, and create a sense of calm.
- *Sleep Aid*: Chamomile is known for its mild sedative effects, which can help individuals struggling with insomnia or difficulty sleeping due to stress. Consuming chamomile tea before bed can promote restful sleep, aiding in overall stress management.
- *Digestive Relief*: Stress and anxiety can lead to digestive issues, and chamomile's anti-inflammatory and antispasmodic properties can help alleviate symptoms such as bloating and indigestion. This can contribute to overall well-being and reduced stress levels.

6.2 Recipes for Stress and Anxiety Relief

(a) Ashwagandha Root Tea for Daily Stress Management

Ingredients:

  1 cup of water

  1 teaspoon of honey (optional)

  1 slice of lemon (optional)

Preparation Steps:

- Heat the water to a boil in a small saucepan.
- After reaching a boil, stir in the Ashwagandha root powder and turn down the heat to maintain a gentle simmer.
- Let it simmer for about 10 minutes, stirring now and then.
- Take the saucepan off the heat and pour the mixture through a strainer into a mug to eliminate any solids.
- Enhance with honey and a slice of lemon to taste, if preferred.

(b) St. John's Wort Tincture for Mood Support

Ingredients:

1 cup dried St. John's Wort flowers

1 cup high-proof alcohol (like vodka or brandy)

A glass jar with a tight-fitting lid

Instructions:

- Fill the glass jar halfway with dried St. John's Wort flowers.
- Pour the alcohol over the flowers, ensuring they are completely submerged.
- Close the jar securely and keep it in a cool, dark location for 4-6 weeks, shaking it daily to mix the contents.
- After 4-6 weeks, strain the mixture into a clean bottle using a fine-mesh strainer or cheesecloth.
- To use, take 10-20 drops (or as recommended by a healthcare professional) 1-3 times daily for mood support.

(c) **Lavender Infused Oil for Topical Application to Promote Relaxation**

Ingredients:

1 cup dried lavender buds

1 cup of a carrier oil (like jojoba or almond oil)

A glass jar with a secure lid

A fine-mesh strainer or cheesecloth

Preparation Steps:

- Fill the glass jar with the dried lavender buds.
- Cover the buds fully by pouring the carrier oil over them.
- Seal the jar tightly and store it in a dark, cool place for 4 to 6 weeks, shaking the jar daily to ensure the ingredients are well mixed.
- Once the infusion period is complete, use a fine-mesh strainer or cheesecloth to filter the oil into a clean bottle.
- For a calming and fragrant effect, apply a small quantity of the lavender-infused oil to areas like your wrists, temples, or neck.

(d) Chamomile and Lavender Tea for Evening Unwinding

Ingredients:

1 teaspoon dried chamomile flowers

1 teaspoon dried lavender buds

1 cup hot water

1 teaspoon honey (optional)

Instructions:

- Place the dried chamomile flowers and lavender buds in a tea infuser or a teapot.
- Pour hot water over the herbs and let them steep for 5-10 minutes.
- Strain the tea into a mug and add honey for sweetness, if desired.
- Enjoy the tea in the evening to help relax and unwind.

6.3 Herbs for Enhancing Mood

(a) Lemon Balm

Lemon balm is a fragrant herb that has been used traditionally to alleviate stress and anxiety. Its calming properties can help lift the mood and reduce feelings of tension.

- *Cognitive Function*: Beyond its mood-enhancing benefits, lemon balm has been shown to improve cognitive function. Studies suggest that it can enhance alertness and memory, making it useful for those dealing with stress-related cognitive impairment.
- *How to Use*: Lemon balm can be consumed as a tea, in supplement form, or used in aromatherapy to promote relaxation and improve mood. See recipe for Green Tea and Lemon Balm Infusion (section 3.6.1).

(b) Rhodiola

Rhodiola is an adaptogenic herb known for its ability to increase energy and combat fatigue. It helps balance stress hormones, making it easier for individuals to cope with daily stressors.

- Combating Fatigue: By supporting the body's stress response, Rhodiola can help reduce feelings of burnout and exhaustion. This makes it particularly useful for individuals experiencing stress-related fatigue.
- How to Use: Rhodiola can be taken as a supplement, typically in capsule form, to help manage stress and support energy levels.

(c) Saffron

Saffron has been studied for its potential to treat mild to moderate depression. Clinical trials have shown that it can be as effective as traditional antidepressants, offering a natural alternative for mood support.

- Mood Enhancement: The herb's ability to increase serotonin levels contributes to its mood-boosting effects. This can help alleviate feelings of sadness and improve overall mental well-being.
- How to Use: Saffron can be consumed as a supplement, in teas, or incorporated into meals, providing a flavorful way to support mood and mental health.

6.4 Recipes for Mood Enhancement

(a) Lemon Balm and Rhodiola Morning Tonic

Ingredients:

1 teaspoon dried lemon balm leaves

1 teaspoon dried Rhodiola root powder

1 cup hot water

1 teaspoon honey (optional)

Instructions:

- Place the lemon balm leaves and Rhodiola root powder in a teapot or tea infuser.
- Pour hot water over the herbs and let them steep for 5-10 minutes.
- Strain the tea into a mug and add honey for sweetness, if desired.
- Drink the tonic in the morning to start the day with a mood boost and energy enhancement.

(b) Saffron and Tulsi Tea for Emotional Uplift

Ingredients:

2-3 saffron strands

1 teaspoon dried Tulsi (Holy Basil) leaves

1 cup hot water

1 teaspoon honey or agave syrup (optional)

Instructions:

- Place the saffron strands and Tulsi leaves in a teapot or tea infuser.
- Pour hot water over the herbs and let them steep for 5-7 minutes.
- Strain the tea into a mug and add honey or agave syrup for sweetness, if desired.
- Enjoy the tea during the day for emotional uplift.

(c) Chamomile Honey Yogurt Parfait

Ingredients:

1 cup Greek yogurt

1 tablespoon dried chamomile flowers

1 tablespoon honey

1/4 cup granola

Fresh berries (optional)

Instructions:

- Heat the honey slightly in a microwave-safe dish until it becomes more liquid.
- Mix the dried chamomile flowers into the warm honey, allowing them to infuse for a few minutes.
- In a serving dish, layer the Greek yogurt, chamomile-infused honey, granola, and berries, alternating until all ingredients are used.
- Enjoy as a calming and mood-boosting breakfast or snack.

(d) Valerian Lavender Sleep Cookies

1/2 cup softened butter

1/2 cup sugar

1 egg

1 teaspoon vanilla extract

1 1/4 cups all-purpose flour

1/4 teaspoon baking powder

1 teaspoon dried lavender buds

1 teaspoon Valerian root powder

Cooking Instructions:

- Preheat your oven to 350°F (175°C) and line a baking sheet with parchment paper.
- In a large mixing bowl, beat together the butter and sugar until the mixture becomes light and fluffy.
- Add the egg and vanilla extract to the creamy butter and sugar mixture.
- In another bowl, combine the flour, baking powder, dried lavender buds, and Valerian root powder.
- Gradually mix the dry ingredients into the wet mixture until a uniform dough forms.
- Drop spoonfuls of dough onto the prepared baking sheet and bake for approximately 10-12 minutes, or until the edges are golden brown.
- Let the cookies cool on the baking sheet before serving as a delightful treat to promote relaxation and sleep.

(e) Ashwagandha Golden Milk

Ingredients:

1 cup almond milk (or milk of your choice)

1 teaspoon Ashwagandha powder

1 teaspoon turmeric powder

1/2 teaspoon ground cinnamon

1 teaspoon honey or maple syrup (optional)

Instructions:

- Heat the milk in a saucepan over medium heat.
- Stir in the Ashwagandha powder, turmeric powder, and ground cinnamon.
- Stir continuously until the mixture is hot and fully combined.
- Pour into a mug and add honey or maple syrup for sweetness, if desired.
- Enjoy as a warming and calming beverage.

(f) Passionflower Magnolia Bark Smoothie

Ingredients:

1 cup almond milk (or milk of your choice)

1/2 cup Greek yogurt

1/2 banana

1 tablespoon dried passionflower

1 teaspoon Magnolia bark powder

1 teaspoon honey (optional)

Instructions:

- Place all ingredients in a blender and blend until smooth.
- Strain the mixture to remove any solid particles, if necessary.
- Pour into a glass and enjoy for a refreshing and calming smoothie.

CHAPTER 7: BOOSTING PHYSICAL ENERGY

This chapter explores the intricate relationship between human vitality and natural remedies. It discusses how physical energy, often seen as the driving force behind our daily activities, can be influenced and enhanced through the use of herbal treatments. In an era where holistic health approaches are gaining traction, understanding the synergy between physical well-being and herbal interventions provides valuable insights into sustainable wellness practices.

7.1 Physical Energy and the metabolic balance

Physical energy, often described as the capacity to perform work, is integral to our daily lives and overall well-being. When there are changes in the body's physical state during physical activities, this is considered physical energy. Examples of physical energy often involve alterations in physical strength or capacity. When examining the role of physical energy, it is crucial to consider its physiological foundations, including metabolic and cellular processes.

Metabolic Processes

Metabolism encompasses the chemical reactions that occur within the body to maintain life. It is divided into two main categories: catabolism and anabolism.

- Catabolism involves breaking down molecules to release energy. During catabolic reactions, complex molecules like carbohydrates, fats, and proteins are degraded into simpler ones, such as glucose and fatty acids. These reactions release the energy stored in chemical bonds, which the body then uses for various functions.

- Anabolism, on the other hand, focuses on building up complex molecules from simpler ones. This process requires energy input. For example, the synthesis of proteins from amino acids and the creation of cellular components are anabolic processes that consume energy.

Together, catabolism and anabolism constitute the metabolic balance that determines how the body stores and expends energy.

Cellular Processes

At the cellular level, the mitochondria play a critical role in energy production through a process known as cellular respiration. This process can be broken down into several stages:

- Glycolysis: This occurs in the cell's cytoplasm and breaks down glucose into pyruvate, producing a small amount of ATP (adenosine triphosphate), the cell's energy currency. Krebs Cycle: Also known as the citric acid cycle, this process takes place in the mitochondria and further breaks down pyruvate into carbon dioxide. The cycle generates electron carriers, which are used in the next stage.

- Electron Transport Chain: This stage occurs in the inner mitochondrial membrane, where the electron carriers donate electrons to create a proton gradient. This particular gradient enables the synthesis of ATP, which stores energy in a form that cells can readily use. The interplay of these cellular processes ensures that the body has a consistent supply of ATP to meet its energy needs. This ATP is then used for various functions, such as muscle contraction, nerve signal transmission, and cellular repair.

Impact of Fatigue on Health

Fatigue can significantly affect daily life and overall health, impacting both physical and mental well-being. Persistent tiredness hampers productivity, concentration, and decision-making, making it difficult to perform routine tasks or meet work obligations. This can lead to increased stress and frustration.

Physically, chronic fatigue can weaken the immune system, making the body more susceptible to illnesses. It can also interfere with sleep quality, creating a cycle of poor rest and low energy. Mentally, fatigue often correlates with mood disorders like depression and anxiety, further diminishing quality of life. Addressing fatigue through lifestyle adjustments, medical intervention, or both is crucial for maintaining health and achieving a balanced, fulfilling life.

7.2 Herbal Interventions: Supporting Energy Production

Herbs have long been used to enhance energy and vitality. Certain herbs possess properties that support energy production, enhance oxygen uptake, and improve nutrient utilization.

Some herbs stimulate energy production at the cellular level. For example, ginseng has been used for centuries in traditional medicine for its energizing properties. It boosts energy by improving cellular metabolism and enhancing the body's response to stress. Similarly, rhodiola helps combat fatigue and increase endurance by optimizing the production of ATP, the body's primary energy molecule.

Oxygen is crucial for cellular respiration, a process vital for energy generation. Cordyceps, a type of medicinal mushroom, has been shown to enhance oxygen uptake and improve aerobic capacity, making it popular among athletes. This herb increases oxygen flow to cells, boosting endurance and stamina.

Efficient nutrient utilization is key to maintaining energy levels. Ashwagandha, a popular adaptogenic herb, helps improve nutrient absorption and balance blood sugar levels, providing steady energy throughout the day. Additionally, maca root is known for enhancing nutrient utilization, particularly in maintaining balanced hormone levels, which can influence energy and mood.

Incorporating these herbs into one's routine, with proper guidance, can provide a natural and effective way to enhance energy, improve endurance, and support overall vitality.

7.2.1. Prominent Energy-Enhancing Herbs

(a) Ginseng

Ginseng, a renowned adaptogenic herb, excels at boosting energy levels and combating fatigue. Its unique properties enhance physical endurance and sharpen mental alertness, making it a favored choice for individuals seeking a natural energy boost. Ginseng works by regulating the body's stress response and improving overall vitality, which contributes to sustained energy levels. Additionally, it enhances physical performance by increasing stamina, making it beneficial for athletes and those leading active lifestyles. Its impact on cognitive function is also notable, as it helps improve focus and clarity, thereby enhancing mental performance. Incorporating ginseng into one's daily routine can be an effective way to enhance both physical and mental energy, supporting a balanced and vibrant lifestyle.

(b) Rhodiola Rosea

Rhodiola Rosea, a prominent adaptogenic herb, is known for its remarkable ability to enhance energy levels and help the body adapt to stress. It plays a key role in boosting physical performance and reducing fatigue, making it a valuable addition to an active lifestyle. Rhodiola Rosea aids in balancing the body's stress response, promoting resilience, and preventing burnout. This herb's benefits extend to improving endurance, which is particularly useful for athletes or anyone with a demanding schedule. Additionally, it helps alleviate mental fatigue, leading to enhanced focus and clarity. Integrating Rhodiola into one's routine can support overall well-being by fostering both physical vitality and mental sharpness, ultimately contributing to sustained energy and improved quality of life.

(c) Ashwagandha

Ashwagandha is celebrated for its adaptogenic qualities, which assist the body in handling stress effectively. This herb is packed with numerous bioactive elements such as alkaloids, lactones, and saponins, all of which are pivotal in delivering its health benefits. Commonly, it is linked to increased energy levels, enhanced mental clarity, and improved physical stamina. Additionally, it is reputed to strengthen the immune system and promote general well-being. Given its capacity to boost energy and endurance, Ashwagandha is a favored choice for individuals seeking to elevate their vitality and cope better with everyday stressors.

(d) Maca Root

Maca root, a Peruvian adaptogenic herb, is renowned for its energy-enhancing qualities, believed to boost stamina and endurance. This is likely due to its rich nutritional profile, which includes vitamins, minerals, amino acids, and beneficial plant compounds. Maca is also considered an adaptogen, helping the body adapt to stress. It is often used to enhance athletic performance, improve mood, and promote general vitality. The unique combination of nutrients and bioactive compounds in maca root contributes to its reputation as a natural energy booster and overall health enhancer.

(e) Green Tea

Green tea is celebrated for its remarkable ability to invigorate, owing to its unique amalgamation of natural components. Its energizing essence primarily emanates from a harmonious blend of moderate caffeine content and the presence of L-theanine, an amino acid. Unlike conventional caffeinated beverages, green tea offers a balanced surge in energy, distinct from coffee.

Caffeine, a renowned stimulant, heightens alertness and concentration by obstructing the inhibitory neurotransmitter adenosine. Consequently, it imparts a stimulating impact on the nervous system. Green tea typically contains a lower caffeine content than coffee, furnishing a gentler yet sustained boost in energy.

L-theanine complements caffeine by augmenting cognitive function and fostering relaxation. This amino acid amplifies the generation of alpha waves in the brain, indicative of a serene yet vigilant mental disposition. The interplay between caffeine and L-theanine in green tea fosters enhanced mental acuity, concentration, and enduring vitality throughout the day.

Additionally, green tea contains catechins, a type of antioxidant that may enhance physical performance by increasing fat oxidation and improving metabolic rate. These catechins can also contribute to improved endurance during physical activities, making green tea an excellent choice for those looking to enhance their energy and performance naturally.

(f) Peppermint

Peppermint, widely known for its invigorating properties, offers prominent energy-enhancing qualities when used as an essential oil or consumed as tea. The active compounds in peppermint, particularly menthol, are primarily responsible for its stimulating effects. Menthol provides a refreshing and cooling sensation that can help clear the mind and promote alertness.

Peppermint essential oil is often used for its stimulating effects. Inhaling peppermint oil or applying it topically can enhance mental clarity and focus, making it a popular choice for improving concentration during work or study. The scent of peppermint has been shown to increase alertness and cognitive performance, likely due to its ability to stimulate the central nervous system.

Drinking peppermint tea (see earlier section 5.5 for recipe) is another way to benefit from its energy-enhancing properties. The natural compounds in peppermint can help alleviate fatigue and boost energy levels by improving blood circulation and oxygen flow. The refreshing flavor and aroma of peppermint contribute to a sense of rejuvenation and mental clarity, making it an excellent choice for those seeking a natural energy boost without the need for caffeine.

Moreover, peppermint's energy-enhancing qualities are complemented by its ability to relieve stress and improve mood. By promoting relaxation while simultaneously increasing alertness, peppermint offers a balanced approach to boosting energy levels and enhancing overall well-being.

(g) Cordyceps

Cordyceps, a renowned Chinese medicinal mushroom, enhances energy due to unique compounds like cordycepin and adenosine. Cordyceps boosts energy by enhancing oxygen utilization in the body and boosting the production of ATP, which is vital for cellular energy. This improved oxygen utilization is especially beneficial during physical activity, making cordyceps a popular supplement among athletes and those looking to enhance their exercise performance. The increased ATP production helps maintain energy levels and prevents fatigue, allowing for sustained physical and mental activity.

Cordyceps also has adaptogenic properties, meaning it helps the body adapt to stress and maintain balance. By reducing stress and boosting energy, cordyceps supports overall vitality and resilience. The herb's anti-inflammatory and antioxidant effects further contribute to its ability to enhance energy by promoting recovery and reducing oxidative stress, which can drain energy levels.

In addition to enhancing physical performance, cordyceps is also known for its potential to improve mental clarity and focus. The increased ATP production and improved blood circulation associated with cordyceps intake can enhance cognitive function, leading to greater alertness and concentration.

(h) Eleuthero (Siberian Ginseng)

Eleuthero, commonly known as Siberian ginseng, is highly regarded for its prominent energy-enhancing qualities. This adaptogenic herb is known for boosting physical endurance and combating fatigue. By helping the body adapt to stress, eleuthero enhances resilience and stamina, making it an ideal choice for those seeking sustained energy levels.

One of the ways in which eleuthero enhances energy is through its influence on mental and physical performance. It helps improve concentration, focus, and cognitive function, which can be particularly beneficial during periods of intense mental activity. Additionally, eleuthero is known to increase physical endurance, which is useful for athletes or individuals engaged in strenuous physical work.

Eleuthero also supports overall vitality by enhancing the body's ability to handle stress. As an adaptogen, it helps maintain balance in the body's systems, which can lead to improved energy and a greater sense of well-being. The herb's ability to regulate stress hormones and support the adrenal glands contributes to its energy-boosting effects, helping to prevent burnout and maintain consistent energy levels throughout the day.

Moreover, eleuthero has antioxidant properties, which aid in protecting the body from oxidative stress and inflammation, further supporting its role in enhancing energy. Its ability to strengthen the immune system also contributes to its overall energy-enhancing qualities, as a healthy immune system is crucial for maintaining vitality and preventing energy-draining illnesses.

(i) Yerba Mate

Yerba mate, a popular South American herb, is well-known for its prominent energy-enhancing qualities, particularly its ability to improve focus and concentration. This herb contains a blend of naturally occurring stimulants, including caffeine, theobromine, and theophylline, which together provide a balanced energy boost without the apprehension often associated with other caffeinated beverages.

The caffeine in yerba mate stimulates the central nervous system, increasing alertness and combating mental fatigue. This can be especially helpful for tasks that require sustained focus or mental effort. Additionally, theobromine and theophylline contribute to a sense of well-being and promote gentle stimulation, helping to improve concentration and maintain mental clarity.

Yerba mate's combination of stimulants not only enhances cognitive function but also boosts physical energy, making it a great choice for people who want to stay active and alert throughout the day. Furthermore, the herb is packed with antioxidants and nutrients that support overall health, contributing to sustained energy levels and enhanced cognitive performance.

(j) Guarana

Guarana, an herb native to the Amazon basin, is renowned for its prominent energy-enhancing qualities and its ability to improve physical performance. The herb's seeds are rich in caffeine, providing a potent natural stimulant that increases alertness and combats fatigue. This caffeine content not only boosts mental clarity but also enhances stamina, making it a popular choice for athletes and those who want to stay active.

Guarana possesses the capability to stimulate the central nervous system, resulting in heightened energy levels and endurance. Moreover, it is recognized for its capacity to augment metabolism and facilitate fat burning, thereby potentially enhancing physical performance.

Beyond its stimulant effects, guarana also contains antioxidants that support overall health, further contributing to its energy-boosting qualities. The herb's combination of stimulating and health-promoting properties makes it a valuable addition to any regimen aimed at enhancing energy and performance.

7.3 Recipes for Energy-Enhancing Herbal Remedies

7.3.1. Teas and Infusions

(a) Ginseng and Ginger Tea

Ingredients:

1 cup of water

1-2 slices of fresh ginger

1 ginseng tea bag or 1 teaspoon of ginseng powder

1 teaspoon of honey (optional)

Instructions:

- Boil Water: Bring 1 cup of water to a boil.
- Add Ginger: Add the ginger slices to the boiling water. Let it simmer for about 5 minutes to extract the flavor.
- Add Ginseng: Add the ginseng tea bag or powder to the water. Let it steep for another 5-7 minutes.
- Strain and Serve: Strain out the ginger and tea bag (if using), and pour the tea into a cup.
- Sweeten (Optional): Add honey to taste if desired.

(b) Rhodiola and Lemon Balm Tea

Ingredients:

1 cup of water

1 teaspoon of dried Rhodiola root or a Rhodiola tea bag

1 teaspoon of dried lemon balm or a lemon balm tea bag

1 teaspoon of honey or lemon (optional)

Instructions:

Boil Water: Bring 1 cup of water to a boil.

- Add Rhodiola and Lemon Balm: Add the dried Rhodiola root and lemon balm to the boiling water or place both tea bags in a cup and pour the boiling water over them.
- Steep: Let the tea steep for about 5-10 minutes.
- Strain and Serve: If using dried herbs, strain out the leaves and roots, then pour the tea into a cup. If using tea bags, simply remove them.
- Sweeten or Add Lemon (Optional): Add honey or a splash of lemon juice to taste.

7.3.2. Tinctures and Supplements

(a) Maca Root Tincture

Ingredients:

Dried maca root powder or chopped maca root

80-proof vodka or brandy

A glass jar with a tight-fitting lid

Instructions:

- Prepare the Jar: Fill a glass jar halfway with either dried maca root powder or chopped maca root.
- Add Alcohol: Pour 80-proof vodka or brandy over the maca root until the jar is nearly full, leaving approximately 1 inch of space from the top.
- Seal and Store: Secure the jar tightly with a lid and vigorously shake it. Place the jar in a cool, dim location for a duration of 4 to 6 weeks, shaking it once per day.
- Strain: Once the designated time has elapsed, strain the tincture through a fine mesh strainer or cheesecloth into another clean jar. Dispose of the solid remnants.
- Store the Tincture: Transfer the strained tincture into a dark glass bottle equipped with a dropper for convenient usage.

- Usage: Consume 1 to 2 droppers of the tincture daily as a supplement to enhance overall vitality. Commence with a smaller dosage and adjust as necessary.

(b) Guarana Capsules

Ingredients:

Guarana seed powder

Empty gelatin or vegetable capsules

Capsule filling manually or by machine (machine is optional, but helpful for efficiency)

Instructions:

- Fill the Capsules: Using a capsule filling machine or by hand, fill the empty capsules with guarana seed powder. Be careful to avoid spilling the powder, as it can be quite stimulating.
- Seal the Capsules: Close the filled capsules securely.
- Store the Capsules: Store the capsules in an airtight container in a cool, dry place.
- Usage: Take 1 to 2 capsules as needed for moments when extra energy is required. It's important to start with a smaller dose to gauge tolerance, as guarana is quite potent.

7.3.3. Smoothies and Nutritional Boosts

(a) Energy Boosting Smoothie:

Ingredients:

1 ripe banana

1 cup of fresh spinach leaves

1 cup of almond milk (or any preferred milk)

1 tablespoon of maca powder

1 tablespoon of honey (optional)

Ice cubes

Instructions:

- Blend Ingredients: Add the banana, spinach, almond milk, maca powder, and honey (if using) to a blender. Blend until smooth.

- Add Ice: Add a few ice cubes to the blender and blend again until the mixture is cold and smooth.
- Serve: Pour the smoothie into a glass and enjoy immediately.
- Benefits: This smoothie is nutrient-rich and energizing. The banana provides natural sweetness and potassium, the spinach adds vitamins and minerals, and the maca powder boosts energy and vitality.

(b) Pre-workout Energizer

Ingredients:

1 teaspoon of guarana powder

1 cup of beetroot juice

1 tablespoon of lemon juice

1 tablespoon of honey (optional)

Ice cubes

Instructions:

- Mix Ingredients: In a glass, combine the guarana powder, beetroot juice, lemon juice, and honey (if using). Stir well until everything is mixed.
- Add Ice: Add a few ice cubes to the glass to chill the drink.
- Serve: Drink this energizer about 30 minutes before your workout for optimal results.

CHAPTER 8: NATURAL CARE FOR SKIN AND HAIR

8.1 Benefits of Using Herbal Remedies and Natural Ingredients for Skin and Hair Care

In the pursuit of holistic well-being, many individuals are turning to herbal remedies and natural ingredients for their skin and hair care routines. These ingredients, often rooted in traditional medicine, offer a host of benefits due to their rich nutrient profiles and gentle nature. Embracing these remedies can not only enhance beauty but also promote overall health.

Benefits for Skin

- *Gentle on Skin*: Herbal remedies and natural ingredients are typically free from synthetic chemicals, making them less likely to cause irritation or allergic reactions. This makes them suitable for sensitive skin types.

- *Nourishing*: Natural ingredients like aloe vera, honey, and coconut oil are rich in vitamins, antioxidants, and moisturizing properties. These elements deeply nourish the skin, promoting a radiant complexion.
- *Anti-inflammatory Properties*: Many herbal ingredients, such as chamomile and calendula, possess anti-inflammatory and soothing properties, which can be beneficial for calming irritated or inflamed skin.
- *Anti-aging Benefits*: Natural ingredients like green tea, vitamin E, and rosehip oil are renowned for their antioxidant properties, helping to combat free radicals and reduce the appearance of wrinkles and fine lines.

Benefits for Hair
- *Strengthening*: Herbal ingredients such as rosemary, amla, and argan oil are known for strengthening hair, promoting growth, and reducing hair fall. These ingredients are rich in vitamins and fatty acids, which nourish the scalp and hair follicles.
- *Hydration*: Natural oils like jojoba and coconut oil provide deep hydration to the hair, combating dryness and split ends while leaving the hair shiny and healthy.
- *Scalp Health*: Ingredients like tea tree oil, neem, and apple cider vinegar have antibacterial and antifungal properties, helping to maintain a healthy scalp environment and prevent dandruff.
- *Environmentally Friendly*: Using herbal remedies and natural ingredients often aligns with environmentally conscious choices, as many commercial hair care products contain chemicals that can be harmful to the environment when washed down the drain.

8.2 Nutritional Needs for Skin and Hair Health

Nutrition plays a critical role in the health and appearance of our skin and hair. Just as a balanced diet contributes to overall health, it also significantly influences the vitality of our skin and hair, impacting factors such as hydration, elasticity, and resilience. Understanding the connection between nutrition and skin and hair health can guide dietary choices that promote a vibrant and youthful appearance.

Nutritional Needs for Skin Health:
- **Vitamins and Antioxidants:** *Vitamins A, C, and E play pivotal roles in maintaining skin health. Vitamin C is essential for producing collagen, which improves skin elasticity and firmness. Vitamin E acts as a powerful antioxidant that shields the skin from oxidative damage, and Vitamin A promotes the regeneration of skin cells. Consuming foods like leafy greens, citrus fruits, and nuts, which are high in these vitamins, is crucial for sustaining a robust skin barrier.*

- *Healthy Fats:* Omega-3 fatty acids, which are found in fish, walnuts, and flaxseeds, have anti-inflammatory properties and help maintain skin hydration. These fats keep the skin elastic and may protect against sun damage, thus minimizing the signs of aging.
- *Hydration:* Staying properly hydrated is vital for skin health. Drinking plenty of water helps eliminate toxins and maintains skin moisture, reducing the chances of dryness and irritation. Foods high in water content, such as cucumbers and watermelon, also aid in hydrating the skin.

Nutritional Needs for Hair Health:

- *Protein:* Since hair is mainly made of keratin, a protein, it is essential to consume adequate protein from sources like lean meats, beans, and dairy to support hair strength and growth. Insufficient protein intake can result in brittle hair and increased hair loss.
- *Vitamins and Minerals:* Key vitamins and minerals are essential for hair vitality. Biotin, a B-vitamin found in eggs, nuts, and whole grains, promotes hair growth and helps prevent hair thinning. Zinc, present in shellfish, nuts, and seeds, is important for maintaining healthy scalp conditions and preventing hair loss.
- *Iron:* Iron deficiency can cause hair loss, especially in women. Eating iron-rich foods such as red meat, spinach, and legumes enhances blood circulation and provides vital nutrients to hair follicles, encouraging robust hair growth.

8.3 Herbal Remedies and Natural Ingredients for Nourishing and Protecting the Skin

Herbal remedies and natural ingredients have been cherished for their nourishing and protective properties, enhancing skin health and providing effective solutions for various skin concerns. Among the many beneficial ingredients, aloe vera, calendula, chamomile, and lavender stand out for their unique properties that contribute to skin well-being. These herbs offer natural solutions for hydration, healing, and soothing, aligning with holistic beauty practices.

8.3.1. Aloe Vera

Aloe vera is renowned for its cooling and calming attributes. The gel derived from its leaves harbors a plethora of vitamins, minerals, and antioxidants, all of which play a role in its skin-nourishing properties. Aloe vera excels in skin hydration, facilitates healing, and diminishes inflammation. It is frequently employed in the treatment of sunburn due to its anti-inflammatory characteristics, which aid in alleviating discomfort and redness. Furthermore, aloe vera's moisturizing capabilities render it advantageous for dry or sensitive skin types.

8.3.2. Calendula

Calendula, also known as marigold, has been used for centuries as a skin remedy. Its bright orange petals contain flavonoids and saponins, which provide anti-inflammatory and antiseptic properties. Calendula is often used in skincare products for its ability to soothe irritated skin, promote healing, and reduce swelling. It is especially beneficial for sensitive or damaged skin, as it helps to calm and rejuvenate. Calendula's gentle nature makes it suitable for various skin types, including delicate baby skin.

8.3.3. Chamomile

Chamomile is known for its calming and soothing properties. The herb contains compounds such as bisabolol and chamazulene, which have anti-inflammatory and antioxidant effects. Chamomile is often used to address skin irritation, redness, and inflammation. It is also beneficial for sensitive skin, as it helps to calm and reduce the risk of allergic reactions. Chamomile's gentle yet effective properties make it an excellent choice for those with easily irritated or reactive skin.

8.3.4. Lavender

Lavender is renowned for its relaxing scent and healing properties. The essential oil extracted from lavender flowers contains linalool and linalyl acetate, which have anti-inflammatory, antifungal, and antibacterial effects. Lavender is often used to soothe skin irritations, promote healing, and balance skin tone. Its calming properties make it a popular ingredient in products designed for stress relief and relaxation. Additionally, lavender's antiseptic qualities help protect the skin from infections, making it useful for treating minor cuts and wounds.

8.4 Herbal Remedies and Natural Ingredients for Promoting Hair Growth, Reducing Hair Loss, and Improving Scalp Health

Herbal remedies and natural ingredients have been used for centuries to promote hair health, offering effective solutions for common issues such as hair loss, slow growth, and poor scalp health. Among the most notable ingredients, rosemary, peppermint, coconut oil, and castor oil stand out for their unique properties that support hair vitality. These herbs and oils provide nourishment, stimulation, and protection, contributing to healthy and vibrant hair.

8.4.1. Rosemary

Rosemary is renowned for its capacity to promote hair growth and enhance scalp well-being. This herb harbors ursolic acid, a compound that boosts blood circulation to the scalp, thereby nourishing hair follicles with vital nutrients. Utilized in the form of oil, rosemary is prized for its ability to bolster hair thickness and counteract hair loss. Furthermore, its antimicrobial attributes aid in sustaining a hygienic scalp environment, warding off dandruff and related scalp issues. Consistent application of rosemary oil or hair products infused with rosemary can contribute to the development of resilient, lustrous hair.

8.4.2. Peppermint

Peppermint is known for its invigorating and refreshing properties. The essential oil extracted from peppermint leaves contains menthol, which stimulates blood circulation to the scalp and encourages hair growth. Peppermint oil also has antifungal and antibacterial effects, making it useful for treating and preventing scalp infections. Additionally, its cooling sensation helps soothe scalp irritation and itching, providing relief for sensitive or inflamed skin. Incorporating peppermint oil into hair care routines can enhance scalp health and support healthy hair growth.

8.4.3. Coconut Oil

Coconut oil is renowned for its moisturizing and protective properties. Rich in fatty acids, especially lauric acid, coconut oil penetrates the hair shaft, providing deep hydration and preventing protein loss. This helps strengthen the hair, reduce breakage, and promote healthy growth. Coconut oil also has antibacterial and antifungal properties, making it effective for maintaining scalp health and preventing dandruff. Its versatility and nourishing effects make it a popular choice for various hair and scalp concerns.

8.4.4. Castor Oil

Castor oil is highly valued for its efficacy in fostering hair growth and enhancing scalp vitality. Packed with ricinoleic acid, this oil facilitates improved blood circulation to the scalp, fostering an environment conducive to hair growth. Furthermore, its abundant reservoir of omega-6 fatty acids provides nourishment to hair follicles, contributing to the development of robust and vibrant hair strands. Moreover, the antibacterial and antifungal properties inherent in castor oil serve as a shield against scalp infections and dandruff. Consistent application of castor oil can yield the desired outcomes of denser, more voluminous hair and a scalp teeming with vitality.

8.5 Homemade Recipes for Skin and Hair using Natural Ingredients

8.5.1. Facial Masks

(a) Hydrating Honey and Avocado Mask

Ingredients:

  1 ripe avocado

  1 tablespoon honey

Instructions:

- Puree the avocado until it's creamy and smooth.
- Stir the honey into the pureed avocado.
- Smooth the mixture over your face and let it sit for 15–20 minutes.
- Wash off with lukewarm water.

(b) Brightening Turmeric and Yogurt Mask

Ingredients:

1 tablespoon plain yogurt

1 teaspoon turmeric powder

Instructions:

- Combine the yogurt and turmeric thoroughly.
- Apply the blend evenly to your face and leave it for 10–15 minutes.
- Remove with cool water.

8.5.2. Toners

(a) Green Tea and Witch Hazel Toner

Ingredients:

1 cup brewed green tea

1/4 cup witch hazel

Instructions:

- Prepare the green tea and allow it to cool.
- Combine the cooled green tea with witch hazel.
- Transfer the mixture to a spray bottle for easy application after washing your face.

(b) Apple Cider Vinegar and Rose Water Toner

Ingredients:

1/2 cup of rose water

2 tablespoons of apple cider vinegar

Instructions:

- Combine the rose water with the apple cider vinegar.
- Transfer the mixture to a spray bottle and apply it following your cleansing routine.

8.5.3. Moisturizers

(a) Aloe Vera and Coconut Oil Moisturizer

Ingredients:

2 tablespoons of aloe vera gel

1 tablespoon of coconut oil

Instructions:

- Blend the aloe vera gel with the coconut oil until smooth.
- Use as a light moisturizer by applying it to the skin.

(b) Shea Butter and Jojoba Oil Moisturizer

Ingredients:

2 tablespoons of shea butter

1 tablespoon of jojoba oil

Instructions:

- Melt the shea butter using a double boiler.
- Mix in the jojoba oil.
- Let it cool and solidify.
- Apply to the skin as needed.

8.5.4. Hair Masks

(a) Banana and Olive Oil Hair Mask

Ingredients:

1 ripe banana

2 tablespoons of olive oil

Instructions:

- Mash the banana until smooth.
- Mix in the olive oil.
- Apply to the hair and scalp, leave on for 20–30 minutes, and rinse thoroughly.

(b) Egg and Yogurt Hair Mask

Ingredients:

1 egg

2 tablespoons of plain yogurt

Instructions:

- Beat the egg.
- Mix in the yogurt.
- Apply to the hair and scalp, leave on for 20–30 minutes, and rinse with cool water.

8.5.5. Scalp Treatments

(a) Tea Tree Oil and Jojoba Oil Treatment

Ingredients:

2 tablespoons of jojoba oil

5 drops of tea tree oil

Instructions:

- Mix the oils together.
- Massage into the scalp and leave on for 15–20 minutes.
- Wash with a mild shampoo.

(b) Apple Cider Vinegar Scalp Rinse

Ingredients:

1/2 cup of apple cider vinegar

1 cup of water

Instructions:

Mix *the apple cider vinegar and water.*

After shampooing, pour the mixture over the scalp and massage gently.

Rinse with cool water.

8.5.6. Hair Rinses

(a) Rosemary Hair Rinse

Ingredients:

1 cup of water

1 tablespoon of dried rosemary

Instructions:

- Boil the water and steep the rosemary for 10–15 minutes.
- Let it cool.
- Pour over the hair after shampooing and leave in or rinse out as desired.

(b) Chamomile Hair Rinse

Ingredients:

1 cup of water

1 tablespoon of dried chamomile flowers

Instructions:

- Boil the water and steep the chamomile flowers for 10–15 minutes.
- Let it cool.
- Pour over the hair after shampooing and leave in or rinse.

CHAPTER 9: ENHANCING COGNITIVE FUNCTIONS

9.1 The Concept of Cognitive Enhancement

Cognitive enhancement refers to the augmentation of cognitive functions, such as memory, attention, creativity, or intelligence, beyond the typical human experience. This pursuit of heightened cognitive abilities is fueled by advancements in neuroscience, pharmacology, and technology, offering new avenues for enhancing mental performance. Cognitive enhancement is commonly defined as interventions in humans aimed at improving mental functioning beyond what is needed to maintain or restore good health (Dresler & Repantis, 2015).

The concept of cognitive enhancement has broad applications, ranging from improving academic performance and workplace productivity to addressing cognitive decline associated with aging or neurological disorders. Common methods of cognitive enhancement include pharmaceuticals (often referred to as nootropics), brain stimulation, brain-training exercises, transcranial direct current stimulation (tDCS), and lifestyle modifications like diet and exercise (Thair et al., 2017).

However, cognitive enhancement is not without its ethical, social, and health-related challenges. The desire for enhanced cognitive abilities raises questions about fairness, access, and the potential long-term effects on health and well-being. Despite these concerns, the growing interest in cognitive enhancement underscores a fundamental human desire to transcend limitations and optimize mental performance, highlighting its relevance in both personal and professional domains (Dresler & Repantis, 2015).

9.2 The Use of Natural Methods to Improve Memory and Mental Speed

In an era defined by rapid technological advancements and increasing cognitive demands, many individuals seek ways to enhance their memory and mental speed. Mental speed is a core attribute of cognitive agents and is crucial for prompt and appropriate responses in complex settings. In psychology and neuroscience, cognitive agents typically refer to humans or animals whose cognitive functions are being studied.

While pharmaceuticals and technological interventions offer potential solutions, natural methods for cognitive enhancement (aided by cognitive agents) have garnered significant attention for their accessibility, safety, and holistic benefits. These methods leverage lifestyle changes, dietary

110

adjustments, physical exercise, and mental training to bolster cognitive function, providing an appealing alternative to synthetic solutions.

Methods for improving cognitive function through natural methods often underscore the importance of adopting lifestyle and dietary habits conducive to brain health. Consuming diets rich in antioxidants, omega-3 fatty acids, and other nutrients beneficial for brain function is linked to improved cognitive abilities and a reduced risk of cognitive decline. Incorporating physical exercise, especially aerobic activities, is also acknowledged for its ability to enhance brain performance by improving blood circulation and promoting neuroplasticity. Additionally, engaging in mental exercises such as mindfulness meditation, puzzles, and memory games proves effective in refining cognitive abilities and fostering mental acuity.

The use of natural methods to improve memory and mental speed aligns with a holistic perspective on health, emphasizing balance and sustainability. These approaches not only enhance cognitive function but also promote overall well-being, making them attractive options for individuals looking to optimize their mental capabilities while maintaining a healthy lifestyle.

9.3 Herbal Remedies and Natural Supplements for Memory and Cognitive Function

Herbal remedies and natural supplements have a long history of being used to enhance memory and cognitive function. Traditional herbs like ginkgo biloba, bacopa monnieri, gotu kola, and ashwagandha are renowned for their cognitive-enhancing properties. These herbs work through various mechanisms, such as increasing cerebral blood flow, enhancing neurotransmitter function, and reducing inflammation, to support brain health.

9.3.1. Ginkgo Biloba: Increasing Cerebral Blood Flow

Ginkgo biloba is a widely used herbal supplement recognized for its capability to enhance blood circulation, particularly within the brain. Rich in flavonoids and terpenoids, it facilitates the dilation of blood vessels, thereby augmenting blood flow to cerebral tissues. This heightened circulation ensures a consistent delivery of oxygen and essential nutrients to the brain, potentially enhancing memory and cognitive function. Moreover, the increased blood flow aids in the removal of metabolic waste products, promoting overall brain health and mitigating the risk of cognitive decline.

9.3.2. Bacopa Monnieri (Brahmi): Enhancing Neurotransmitter Function

Bacopa monnieri, commonly known as Brahmi, is celebrated for its cognitive-enhancing effects, primarily through its influence on neurotransmitters. Bacopa contains compounds called bacosides, which enhance the function of acetylcholine, a neurotransmitter associated with memory and learning. This herb also influences serotonin and dopamine, which contribute to mood regulation and cognitive processes. By optimizing neurotransmitter function, bacopa monnieri supports improved memory, focus, and mental clarity.

9.3.3. Gotu Kola and Ashwagandha: Reducing Inflammation

Gotu kola and ashwagandha are herbs known for their anti-inflammatory properties, which are crucial for brain health. Gotu kola contains triterpenoids, which have anti-inflammatory and antioxidant effects. Chronic inflammation in the brain can impair cognitive function and contribute to neurodegenerative diseases, so reducing inflammation is vital for maintaining cognitive health. Ashwagandha, an adaptogenic herb, also possesses anti-inflammatory properties and helps reduce oxidative stress, which can damage brain cells. By reducing inflammation and protecting against oxidative damage, these herbs support cognitive longevity and improve mental clarity.

9.4 Recipes for Cognitive Enhancement

(a) Ginkgo Biloba and Matcha Energy Balls

Ingredients:
1 cup of pitted dates
1/2 cup of nuts (e.g., almonds or cashews)
2 teaspoons of matcha powder
1 teaspoon of ginkgo biloba powder
1 tablespoon of honey
1/4 teaspoon of vanilla extract
1/4 teaspoon of sea salt

Instructions:

- Combine the dates and nuts in a food processor, blending until a dough-like texture is achieved.

- Incorporate matcha powder, ginkgo biloba powder, honey, vanilla extract, and sea salt into the food processor, blending until thoroughly integrated.
- Shape the mixture into small balls by scooping out portions.
- Chill the energy balls in the refrigerator for a minimum of one hour before serving.

(b) Gotu Kola Salad with Citrus Dressing

Ingredients:

1 cup of gotu kola leaves, finely chopped

1 cup of mixed salad greens

1 orange, peeled and segmented

1/4 cup of crumbled feta cheese

2 tablespoons of olive oil

1 tablespoon of orange juice

1 teaspoon of honey

1/4 teaspoon of salt

1/4 teaspoon of black pepper

Instructions:

- Mix gotu kola leaves, assorted salad greens, orange segments, and crumbled feta cheese in a spacious bowl.
- In a separate container, blend olive oil, freshly squeezed orange juice, honey, salt, and pepper to create the dressing.
- Drizzle the dressing over the salad mixture and delicately toss until evenly coated.

(c) Bacopa Monnieri Herbal Tea

Ingredients:

2 teaspoons of dried bacopa monnieri leaves

1 cup of hot water

Honey or lemon, to taste

Instructions:

- Place the dried bacopa monnieri leaves in a tea infuser or tea bag.
- Pour hot water over the leaves and let it steep for 5–7 minutes.
- Remove the infuser or tea bag and add honey or lemon to taste, if desired.

(d) Bacopa Monnieri Blueberry Overnight Oats

Ingredients:

1/2 cup of rolled oats

1/2 cup of almond milk

1/4 cup of fresh blueberries

1 tablespoon of honey

1/2 teaspoon of bacopa monnieri powder

1/4 teaspoon of vanilla extract

1 tablespoon of chopped nuts (optional)

Instructions:

- In a mason jar or container, combine the rolled oats, almond milk, blueberries, honey, bacopa monnieri powder, and vanilla extract.
- Mix well and cover the jar. Refrigerate overnight or for at least 4 hours.
- In the morning, top with chopped nuts if desired, and enjoy.

(e) Gotu Kola Avocado Toast

Ingredients:

2 slices of whole grain bread

1 ripe avocado

1/4 cup of gotu kola leaves, finely chopped

1 tablespoon of olive oil

1/2 teaspoon of lemon juice

1/4 teaspoon of salt

1/4 teaspoon of black pepper

1/4 teaspoon of chili flakes (optional)

Instructions:

- Toast the slices of bread to your liking.

- In a bowl, mash the avocado and mix it with the gotu kola leaves, olive oil, lemon juice, salt, and black pepper.
- Spread the avocado mixture on the toasted bread.
- Sprinkle with chili flakes, if desired, and serve immediately.

CHAPTER 10: HERBAL REMEDIES AND NATURAL RECIPES FOR SPECIFIC HEALTH CONDITIONS

Herbs have long been a cornerstone in managing a diverse array of health issues, including heart problems, diabetes, inflammation, muscle and joint pain, as well as kidney and liver diseases. Their use extends to treating gastrointestinal and respiratory diseases, gastritis, cholesterol imbalances, gallbladder and pancreas issues, and even seasonal ailments like colds and flu. Additionally, herbs play a role in addressing hormonal imbalances, metabolic diseases, and weight control. There are also specific herbal remedies and recipes for headaches. Scientific research continues to support and validate the benefits of these traditional herbal approaches, confirming their effectiveness and expanding our understanding of their properties.

10.1 Cardiovascular diseases: Herbs and Natural Remedies

Key herbs known for their cardioprotective properties include:

1) Hawthorn (Crataegus spp.): Often referred to as the "heart herb," hawthorn is widely used to support heart health. It contains antioxidants such as flavonoids and oligomeric proanthocyanidins, which help improve blood flow, strengthen blood vessels, and normalize blood pressure. Hawthorn can also reduce angina and enhance cardiac function.

2) Garlic (Allium sativum): Garlic is renowned for its ability to lower cholesterol and blood pressure. Allicin, its active compound, has anti-inflammatory properties and can improve overall heart health by reducing the risk of atherosclerosis.

3) Ginger (Zingiber officinale): Ginger possesses anti-inflammatory and antioxidant effects that benefit cardiovascular health. It helps improve circulation and reduce cholesterol levels, contributing to better heart function.

4) Cayenne Pepper (Capsicum annuum): Cayenne pepper contains capsaicin, which can enhance circulation, lower blood pressure, and reduce cholesterol. It's often used to stimulate the cardiovascular system and can help prevent heart attacks.

5) Ginkgo Biloba: Ginkgo biloba is known for its ability to improve circulation and support heart health. Its antioxidant properties help prevent oxidative damage, while its vasodilatory effects enhance blood flow and reduce the risk of clots.

6) Motherwort (Leonurus cardiaca): This herb is aptly named for its heart benefits. Motherwort has calming properties and is often used to treat heart palpitations and anxiety-related heart issues. It also helps regulate heart rhythm.

7) Turmeric (Curcuma longa): Turmeric boasts curcumin, renowned for its robust anti-inflammatory and antioxidant attributes. It aids in enhancing endothelial function, pivotal for maintaining heart health, while mitigating inflammation linked to cardiovascular ailments.

(a) Hawthorn Berry Tincture: See Chapter 4

(b) Garlic and Lemon Tonic: See Chapter 4

(c) Garlic Tincture

Ingredients:

Fresh garlic cloves

Apple cider vinegar

Instructions:

- Peel and crush fresh garlic cloves.
- Place the crushed garlic in a glass jar.
- Cover the garlic with apple cider vinegar.
- Seal the jar and let it sit for 2 weeks, shaking it daily.
- Strain the garlic and store the liquid in a dark glass bottle.
- Usage: Take 1-2 drops in water daily.

(d) Motherwort Tincture

Ingredients:

Dried motherwort

Vodka (40% alcohol)

Instructions:

- Fill a glass jar halfway with dried motherwort herb.
- Pour vodka over the herb until it is completely submerged.

- Seal the jar tightly and allow it to steep for 4-6 weeks, shaking periodically.
- After the steeping period, strain the liquid and transfer it to a dark-colored bottle for storage.
- Directions for use: Dilute 20-30 drops of the tincture in water, and consume up to three times a day.

(e) Dandelion Root Tea

Ingredients:
Dried dandelion root
Water

Instructions:
- Boil 1 cup of water.
- Add 1 teaspoon of dried dandelion root.
- Let it steep for 5-10 minutes, then strain.
- Usage: Drink once daily.

(f) Ginger-Garlic Elixir

Ingredients:
Fresh ginger
Fresh garlic
Honey
Apple cider vinegar
Instructions:
- Blend equal parts of ginger and garlic.
- Mix with honey and apple cider vinegar to taste.
- Store in a glass jar.
- Usage: Take 1 teaspoon daily.

(g) Turmeric and Black Pepper Capsules

Ingredients:
Ground turmeric

Ground black pepper

Empty capsules

Instructions:

Mix 1-part black pepper with 10 parts turmeric.

Fill empty capsules with the mixture.

Usage: Take 1-2 capsules daily.

(h) Ginkgo Biloba Extract

Ingredients:

Dried ginkgo biloba leaves

Vodka (40% alcohol)

Instructions:

- Begin by filling a glass jar halfway with dried ginkgo biloba leaves.
- Pour vodka over the leaves until they are completely submerged.
- Seal the jar tightly and allow it to steep for 4-6 weeks, remembering to give it an occasional shake.
- Once the steeping period is complete, strain the liquid and transfer it into a dark bottle for storage.
- Directions for use: Dilute 20-40 drops of the tincture in water, and consume daily.

(i) Green Tea Extract

Ingredients:

High-quality green tea extract capsules or green tea leaves

Instructions:

- If using green tea leaves: Steep the green tea leaves in hot water for 3-5 minutes.
- If using green tea extract capsules: Follow the dosage instructions on the packaging.

- Usage: Drink one cup of brewed green tea daily or take the green tea extract capsules as directed on the package.

(j) Pomegranate Extract

Ingredients:

Fresh pomegranates

Instructions:
- Cut the pomegranates in half and remove the seeds.
- Place the seeds in a juicer to extract the juice. If you don't have a juicer, you can also use a blender; just pulse the seeds lightly and then strain the mixture to collect the juice.
- Pour the juice into a saucepan and bring it to a simmer over low heat, stirring occasionally until it turns into a thicker, more potent extract.
- Cool and Store.
- Usage: Add a few teaspoons of the pomegranate extract to water, tea, or any beverage of choice.

(k) Omega-3 Fish Oil Supplements

Instructions:
Purchase high-quality fish oil capsules.
Usage: Follow the dosage instructions on the packaging.

10.2 Herbs for Lowering Cholesterol Levels
Herbs commonly used to help manage cholesterol levels include:
1) Garlic - Contains compounds that may help lower LDL or ow-density lipoprotein (bad cholesterol) and raise HDL or high-density lipoprotein (good cholesterol).
2) Turmeric - Contains curcumin, which has anti-inflammatory properties and may help lower cholesterol levels.
3) Guggul - Extract from the guggul tree has been traditionally used to lower cholesterol and triglycerides.
4) Fenugreek - Seeds contain soluble fiber, which can help lower cholesterol.
5) Artichoke Leaf - May increase bile production, aiding in the breakdown of cholesterol.
6) Ginger - May help reduce cholesterol and improve heart health.

7) Green Tea - Contains catechins that may help lower LDL cholesterol.

8) Flaxseed - High in fiber and omega-3 fatty acids, which can help lower cholesterol.

9) Hawthorn - Contains compounds that may lower cholesterol and improve heart health.

10) Psyllium - A soluble fiber that helps lower cholesterol by binding with bile acids.

10.2. High Cholesterol: Herbs and Natural Remedies

(a) Oatmeal with Flaxseed and Berries

Ingredients:

1 cup of oatmeal

1 tablespoon of ground flaxseed

1/2 cup of mixed berries

1 cup of water or milk

Instructions:

- Cook oatmeal with water or milk as per package instructions.
- Mix in ground flaxseed and top with mixed berries.
- Usage: Enjoy for breakfast.

(b) Salmon and Walnut Salad

Ingredients:

Grilled or baked salmon fillet

Mixed salad greens

1/4 cup of chopped walnuts

Olive oil and lemon dressing

Instructions:

- Prepare the salad with mixed greens and chopped walnuts.
- Top with the grilled or baked salmon.
- Drizzle with olive oil and lemon dressing.
- Usage: Eat for lunch or dinner.

(c) Barley and Bean Soup

Ingredients:

1/2 cup of barley

1 cup of mixed beans

4 cups of vegetable broth

Chopped vegetables (carrots, celery, onions)

Instructions:

- Cook the barley and mixed beans separately.
- In a large pot, sauté chopped vegetables.
- Add vegetable broth, cooked barley, and beans.
- Simmer for 20 minutes.
- Usage: Serve as a meal.

(d) Almond and Plant Sterol-Enriched Margarine Spread

Ingredients:

1/4 cup of chopped almonds

1/2 cup of plant sterol-enriched margarine

Instructions:

- Mix chopped almonds into the margarine.
- Spread on whole grain toast or use as a dip.
- Usage: Use as a spread.

(e) Avocado and Whole Grain Bread Toast

Ingredients:

1 ripe avocado

2 slices of whole grain bread

Salt and pepper

Instructions:

- Mash the avocado and spread it on toasted bread slices.
- Season with salt and pepper.
- Usage: Enjoy for breakfast or as a snack.

(f) Grilled Mackerel with Herb Sauce

Ingredients:

Grilled mackerel fillets

Fresh herbs (parsley, basil, etc.)

Olive oil and lemon juice

Instructions:

- Grill the mackerel fillets.
- Mix olive oil and lemon juice with chopped herbs.
- Pour the herb sauce over the grilled mackerel.
- Usage: Serve as a meal.

(g) Psyllium Husk Smoothie

Ingredients:

1 cup of low-fat yogurt

1 tablespoon of psyllium husk

1/2 cup of mixed berries

Instructions:

- Blend all ingredients until smooth.
- Usage: Drink as a snack or meal.

(h) Lentil and Vegetable Stew

Ingredients:

1 cup of lentils

4 cups of vegetable broth

Chopped vegetables (carrots, celery, onions)

Instructions:

- Cook the lentils separately.
- In a large pot, sauté chopped vegetables.
- Add vegetable broth and cooked lentils.
- Add toasted cumin and turmeric powder (I teaspoon each)
- Simmer for 20 minutes.
- Usage: Serve as a meal.

(i) Garlic-Roasted Chickpeas

Ingredients:

1 can of chickpeas

2 tablespoons of olive oil

2-3 garlic cloves, minced

Instructions:

- Drain and rinse the chickpeas.
- Toss them with olive oil and minced garlic.
- Roast in the oven at 400°F (200°C) for 20 minutes.
- Usage: Eat as a snack or add to salads.

(j) Stanol-Fortified Orange Juice Smoothie

Ingredients:

1 cup of stanol-fortified orange juice

1/2 cup of mixed berries

Instructions:

- Blend all ingredients until smooth.
- Usage: Drink as a snack or breakfast drink.

10.3 Herbs for Diabetes

Herbs used for diabetes include:

1) Cinnamon - Known to potentially enhance insulin sensitivity, aiding in the regulation of blood sugar levels.
2) Fenugreek - Contains soluble fiber, which can help control blood sugar levels.
3) Bitter Melon - May mimic insulin and help regulate blood sugar levels.
4) Ginseng - Known for potentially improving insulin sensitivity.
5) Berberine - An alkaloid found in several plants that may lower blood sugar levels.
6) Aloe Vera - Has shown promise in aiding individuals with diabetes by potentially improving blood sugar levels.
7) Ginger - Has been associated with potentially enhancing insulin sensitivity and reducing blood sugar levels.
8) Neem - Known for its blood sugar-lowering properties.
9) Holy Basil - May reduce blood sugar and cholesterol levels.
10) Milk Thistle - Contains silymarin, which may help regulate blood sugar.

10.3.1. Remedies and Natural Recipes for Diabetes

Following are some recipes for managing diabetes:

(a) Cinnamon and Clove Tea

Ingredients:

1 cinnamon stick

2-3 whole cloves

2 cups of water

Directions:

- Bring 2 cups of water to a boil.
- Add the cinnamon stick and cloves to the boiling water.
- Allow the mixture to simmer for approximately 10 minutes.
- Strain the liquid and serve. Enjoy!

(b) Fenugreek Water (Soaked Seeds)

Ingredients:

1 tablespoon of fenugreek seeds

1 cup of water

Instructions:

- Leave 1 tablespoon of fenugreek seeds in 1 cup of water to soak overnight.
- Consume the water first thing in the morning on an empty stomach.
- Recommended frequency: Daily.

(c) Bitter Melon Juice

Ingredients:

1 bitter melon

1 lemon

Water (optional)

Instructions:

- Extract the seeds from the bitter melon and puree the flesh.
- Filter the pureed mixture with ½ cup of water.
- Incorporate lemon juice and salt, then thoroughly stir the juice.

(d) Ginseng Tea

Ingredients:

Dried ginseng root

Water

Instructions:

- Boil 1 cup of water.
- Add 1 teaspoon of dried ginseng root.
- Steep for 5 minutes and strain.

(e) Berberine Tea (Made from Barberry or Goldenseal)

Ingredients:

1 teaspoon of dried barberry or goldenseal

1 cup of water

Instructions:

Boil 1 cup of water.

Add the dried herb and let it steep for 10 minutes.

Strain and drink.

(f) Aloe Vera Smoothie

Ingredients:

2 tablespoons of aloe vera gel

1 cup of water or juice

1 banana (optional)

Instructions:

- Blend all ingredients together.
- Serve chilled.

(g) Bilberry Tea

Ingredients:

1 teaspoon of dried bilberry leaves

1 cup of water

Instructions:

- Boil 1 cup of water.
- Add dried bilberry leaves and let it steep for 5 minutes.
- Strain and drink.

(h) Nopal Salad

Ingredients:

Nopal cactus paddles

Tomato

Onion

Cilantro

Lime juice

Olive oil

Instructions:
- Clean and dice the nopal paddles.
- Boil for 10 minutes and drain.
- Mix with chopped tomatoes, onions, cilantro, lime juice, and olive oil.

(i) Turmeric and Black Pepper Capsules

See recipe used to manage heart problems,

(j) Ginger Lemon Honey Tea

Ingredients:

Fresh ginger

Lemon juice

Honey

Water

Instructions:
- Boil 1 cup of water.
- Add grated ginger and let it steep for 5 minutes.
- Add lemon juice and honey to taste.
- Strain and serve.

(k) Garlic Infused Olive Oil

Ingredients:

Fresh garlic cloves

Olive oil

Instructions:

- Crush a few garlic cloves.
- Heat olive oil and add the garlic.
- Let it simmer for 10 minutes, then cool and strain.
- Store in a glass bottle.
- Usage: Use as a dressing or in cooking.

(l) Holy Basil (Tulsi) Tea

Ingredients:

Fresh or dried holy basil leaves

Water

Instructions:

- Boil 1 cup of water.
- Add a few fresh or dried holy basil leaves.
- Steep for 5 minutes and strain.

(m) Neem Infusion

Ingredients:

Fresh or dried neem leaves

Water

Instructions:

- Boil 1 cup of water.
- Add a few fresh or dried neem leaves.
- Steep for 5-10 minutes and strain.

(n) Milk Thistle Tea

Ingredients:

Dried milk thistle seeds

Water

Instructions:

- Crush 1 teaspoon of dried milk thistle seeds.
- Boil 1 cup of water.
- Add the seeds and let it steep for 5 minutes.
- Strain and drink.

10.3. Inflammation, Muscle and Joint Pain: Herbs and Natural Remedies

Herbs:

1) Turmeric - Contains curcumin, well-known for its powerful anti-inflammatory properties.
2) Ginger - Acknowledged for its capacity to diminish inflammation and relieve discomfort.
3) Boswellia - Also known as Indian frankincense, helps reduce inflammation and pain.
4) Devil's Claw - Traditionally used to treat joint pain and inflammation.
5) Willow Bark - Contains salicin, a compound akin to aspirin, effective in easing pain.
6) Peppermint - Provides a cooling sensation and can relieve muscle pain.
7) Eucalyptus - Has anti-inflammatory properties and provides pain relief.
8) Arnica - Used topically to relieve muscle soreness and joint pain.
9) St. John's Wort - Noted for its anti-inflammatory and pain-relieving qualities.
10) Rosemary - Contains compounds that reduce inflammation and relieve pain.
11) Capsaicin - Traditionally used to treat inflammation, muscle, and joint pain.

(a) Turmeric and Ginger Tea

Ingredients:

1 tsp grated ginger

1 tsp turmeric powder

2 cups water

Honey (if desired)

Instructions:

- Boil 2 cups of water in a pot.

- Add grated ginger and turmeric powder to the boiling water.
- Simmer the mixture for 5-10 minutes.
- Strain the liquid and sweeten with honey if you like.

(b) Cherry Juice (for arthritis, joint pain)

Ingredients:

Fresh cherries or cherry juice concentrate

Instructions:

- Blend fresh cherries or use cherry juice concentrate.
- Add water if needed.

(c) Banana Smoothie with Spinach and Yogurt

Ingredients:

1 banana

1 cup of spinach

1 cup of yogurt

1 cup of milk or water

Instructions:

- Blend all ingredients until smooth.
- Chill and serve.

(d) Cayenne and Coconut Oil Salve

Ingredients:

1 tablespoon of cayenne pepper

1/2 cup of coconut oil

Few drops of essential oil (of your choice)

Instructions:

- Mix cayenne pepper and coconut oil.
- Heat gently until well mixed.
- Add a few drops of essential oil after removing from heat
- Cool and store in a glass jar.
- Apply sparingly to affected areas to relieve pain and improve circulation. Test on a small area first. Avoid broken skin.

(e) Arnica Infused Oil

Ingredients:
1 cup of dried arnica flowers
1 cup of olive oil

Instructions:
- Place arnica flowers in a glass jar.
- Cover with olive oil.
- Let it sit for 2 weeks, shaking occasionally.
- Strain and store.
- Usage: Apply to sore muscles.

(f) Epsom Salt Bath

Ingredients:
2 cups of Epsom salt
Warm bath water

Instructions:
- Add Epsom salt to warm bath water.
- Soak for 20 minutes before bath.

(g) Peppermint and Eucalyptus Rub

Ingredients:
1/2 cup of coconut oil

10 drops of peppermint essential oil

10 drops of eucalyptus essential oil

Instructions:

- Mix all ingredients together.
- Store in a glass jar.
- Usage: Rub on sore muscles.

(h) Rosemary and Olive Oil Massage Blend

Ingredients:

1/2 cup of olive oil

10 drops of rosemary essential oil

Instructions:

- Mix olive oil and rosemary essential oil.
- Store in a glass bottle.
- Usage: Use as a massage oil.

(i) Turmeric Golden Milk

Ingredients:

1 cup of milk (or plant-based alternative)

1 teaspoon of turmeric powder

1/2 teaspoon of ground ginger

Honey (optional)

Instructions:

- Warm the milk.
- Add turmeric and ginger.
- Stir until well mixed.
- Sweeten with honey if desired.
- Usage: Drink before bedtime.

(j) Boswellia Tea

Ingredients:

1 teaspoon of dried boswellia

1 cup of water

Instructions:

- Boil 1 cup of water.
- Add boswellia and let it steep for 10 minutes.
- Strain and drink.

(k) Willow Bark Decoction

Ingredients:

1 tablespoon of dried willow bark

1 cup of water

Instructions:

- Boil 1 cup of water.
- Add willow bark and let it simmer for 10 minutes.
- Strain and drink.

(l) Devil's Claw Tincture

Ingredients:

Dried devil's claw root

Vodka (40% alcohol)

Instructions:

- Place dried devil's claw root in a glass jar.
- Cover with vodka and let it sit for 4-6 weeks, shaking occasionally.
- Strain and store in a dark bottle.
- Usage: Take 20-30 drops in water daily.

(m) Eucalyptus Oil Blend

Ingredients:

1/2 cup of olive oil

10 drops of eucalyptus essential oil

Instructions:

- Mix olive oil and eucalyptus essential oil.
- Store in a glass bottle.
- Usage: Use as a massage oil or inhalant.

(n) Homemade Capsaicin Cream

Ingredients:

1 teaspoon of cayenne pepper

1/2 cup of coconut oil

Instructions:

- Mix cayenne pepper and coconut oil.
- Warm gently until well mixed.
- Cool and store in a glass jar.
- Usage: Apply to sore areas, avoiding broken skin.

10.4 Kidney and Liver Diseases: herbs and remedies

1) Dandelion Root - Promotes liver health by supporting detoxification and bile production.
2) Nettle Leaf - Acts as a diuretic, helping to flush out toxins and excess fluids.
3) Parsley - A natural diuretic that can aid kidney function and detoxification.
4) Cranberry - Helps prevent urinary tract infections and supports kidney health.
5) Milk Thistle - Contains silymarin, which protects the liver and promotes regeneration.
6) Burdock Root - Supports liver function and helps in detoxification.
7) Licorice Root - Protects the liver and helps with inflammation.

8) Artichoke - Supports liver function and increases bile production.

9) Mint - Aids digestion and may help with liver and kidney function.

10) Lemon Balm - Supports liver health and helps reduce stress.

11) Turmeric - Contains curcumin, well-known for its powerful anti-inflammatory properties.

12) Ginger - Helps with digestion and supports liver health.

(a) Dandelion Root Tea

See recipe under the section on heart diseases.

(b) Nettle Leaf Infusion

Ingredients:

1 tablespoon of dried nettle leaves

1 cup of water

Instructions:

- Boil 1 cup of water.
- Add dried nettle leaves.
- Steep for 10-15 minutes.
- Strain and drink.

(c) Parsley Water

Ingredients:

1 handful of fresh parsley

2 cups of water

Instructions:

- Boil 2 cups of water.
- Add fresh parsley.
- Let it simmer for 10 minutes.

- Strain and drink.

(d) Cranberry Juice

Ingredients:

Fresh cranberries or cranberry juice concentrate

Instructions:
- Blend fresh cranberries or use cranberry juice concentrate.
- Add water if needed.
- Strain and use.

(e) Milk Thistle Tea

See recipe under recipes for managing diabetes.

(f) Burdock Root Decoction

Ingredients:

1 tablespoon of dried burdock root

2 cups of water

Instructions:
- Boil 2 cups of water.
- Add dried burdock root and simmer for 10 minutes.
- Strain and drink.

(g) Licorice Root Tea

Ingredients:

1 teaspoon of dried licorice root

1 cup of water

Instructions:

- Boil 1 cup of water.

- Add dried licorice root and steep for 5 minutes.

- Strain and drink.

(i) Artichoke Tea

Ingredients:

Fresh or dried artichoke leaves

1 cup of water

Instructions:

- Boil 1 cup of water.

- Add fresh or dried artichoke leaves.

- Steep for 5-10 minutes.

- Strain and drink.

(j) Dandelion and Mint Detox Tea

Ingredients:

1 tablespoon of dried dandelion root

1 tablespoon of fresh mint leaves

2 cups of water

Instructions:

- Boil 2 cups of water.

- Add dried dandelion root and simmer for 10 minutes.

- Add fresh mint leaves and steep for 5 minutes.

- Strain and drink.

(k) Nettle and Berry Antioxidant Smoothie

Ingredients:

1 cup of fresh or frozen mixed berries

1 tablespoon of dried nettle leaves

1 cup of water or juice

1 banana (optional)

Instructions:
- Blend all ingredients until smooth.
- Usage: Drink as a meal or snack.

(l) Parsley and Cucumber Cleansing Juice

Ingredients:
1 handful of fresh parsley
1 cucumber
1 cup of water or juice

Instructions:
- Blend all ingredients until smooth and serve.

(m) Cranberry Liver Detox Drink

Ingredients:
Fresh cranberries or cranberry juice concentrate
1 tablespoon of lemon juice
1 cup of water

Instructions:
- Blend all ingredients until smooth and drink.

(n) Milk Thistle and Lemon Balm Tea

Ingredients:
1 teaspoon of dried milk thistle seeds
1 tablespoon of fresh lemon balm leaves
1 cup of water

Instructions:

- Bring 1 cup of water to a boil.
- Add the dried milk thistle seeds and simmer for 5 minutes.
- Then, add the fresh lemon balm leaves and steep for an additional 5 minutes.
- Strain the mixture and enjoy your herbal infusion.

(o) Turmeric and Ginger Liver Flush

Ingredients:

1 teaspoon of grated ginger

1 teaspoon of turmeric powder

1 cup of water

Instructions:

- Start by boiling 1 cup of water.
- Add grated ginger and turmeric powder to the boiling water.
- Allow the mixture to simmer for about 5 minutes.
- Strain the infusion and enjoy your ginger-turmeric tea.

(p) Artichoke and Chicory Coffee Substitute

Ingredients:

Dried artichoke leaves

Dried chicory root

Water

Instructions:

- Roast the dried artichoke leaves and chicory root until dark brown.
- Grind the roasted leaves and root into a powder.
- Boil water and add the powder to steep for 5-10 minutes.
- Strain and drink as a coffee substitute.

1) Peppermint - Helps soothe the stomach and relieve symptoms of indigestion, gas, and bloating.

2) Ginger - Eases nausea and improves digestion, often used for morning sickness and motion sickness.

3) Chamomile - Calms the stomach and can help with indigestion, gas, and cramping.

4) Fennel - Relieves bloating, gas, and stomach cramps; also helps with digestion.

5) Licorice Root - Contains compounds that protect the stomach lining and improve digestion.

6) Slippery Elm - Forms a soothing coating over the stomach and intestines, helpful for heartburn and ulcers.

7) Marshmallow Root - Similar to slippery elm, it coats the stomach lining and helps with irritation.

8) Aloe Vera - Soothes the stomach and helps with acid reflux and ulcers.

9) Dandelion Root - Stimulates digestion and may help with indigestion.

10) Turmeric - Contains curcumin, well-known for its powerful anti-inflammatory properties

(a) *Peppermint Ginger* Tea

Ingredients:

1 teaspoon of dried peppermint leaves

1 teaspoon of grated ginger

1 cup of water

Instructions:

- Boil 1 cup of water.
- Add peppermint leaves and ginger.
- Let it steep for 5-10 minutes.
- Strain and drink.

(b) Fennel and Licorice Root Tea

Ingredients:

1 teaspoon of fennel seeds

1 teaspoon of dried licorice root

1 cup of water

Instructions:

- Boil 1 cup of water.
- Add fennel seeds and licorice root.
- Let it steep for 10 minutes.
- Strain and drink.

(c) Aloe Vera Smoothie

Please refer to the recipe provided in the diabetes section.

(d) Probiotic Yogurt and Banana Blend

Ingredients:

1 cup of plain probiotic yogurt

1 banana

Instructions:

- Blend yogurt and banana together until smooth.
- Usage: Eat as a snack or meal.

(e) Apple Cider Vinegar and Honey Drink

Ingredients:

1 tablespoon of apple cider vinegar

1 tablespoon of honey

1 cup of warm water

Instructions:

- Mix all ingredients together until honey dissolves.
- Usage: Drink before meals.

(f) Chamomile Lavender Infusion

Ingredients:

1 teaspoon of dried chamomile flowers

1 teaspoon of dried lavender flowers

1 cup of water

Instructions:

- Boil 1 cup of water.
- Add chamomile and lavender.
- Let it steep for 5-10 minutes.
- Strain and drink.
- Usage: Drink before bed.

(g) Slippery Elm Porridge

Ingredients:

1 tablespoon of slippery elm powder

1 cup of warm water or milk

Honey or sweetener (optional)

Instructions:

- Mix slippery elm powder with warm water or milk.
- Sweeten with honey if desired.
- Usage: Eat once daily.

(h) Papaya Pineapple Digestive Smoothie

Ingredients:

1 cup of fresh papaya

1 cup of fresh pineapple

1 cup of water or juice

Instructions:

- Blend all ingredients until smooth.

(i) Dandelion Root Digestive Tea

Please refer to the recipe provided in the section on managing heart diseases.

(j) Golden Turmeric Milk

Please refer to the recipe provided in the inflammation, muscle, and joint pain section.

10.7 Gallbladder Issues: Herbs and Natural Remedies

1) Milk Thistle - Contains silymarin, which may help support liver and gallbladder health.
2) Dandelion - Stimulates bile production, which can aid in gallbladder function.
3) Artichoke - Helps increase bile production and improve digestion.
4) Turmeric - Contains curcumin, which has anti-inflammatory properties and may support gallbladder health.
5) Peppermint - Can help relieve gallbladder pain and improve digestion.
6) Ginger - Aids in digestion and may help with gallbladder issues.
7) Lemon Balm - Soothes the digestive system and may alleviate gallbladder discomfort.

(a) Milk Thistle Tea

See recipe under recipes for managing diabetes.

(b) Dandelion Root Detox Tea

See recipe used for managing heart disease.

(c) Peppermint Digestive Tea

See recipe under peppermint ginger tea for gastrointestinal diseases.

(d) Turmeric and Honey Drink

Ingredients:

1 teaspoon of turmeric powder

1 cup of warm water or milk

1 tablespoon of honey

Instructions:

- Mix turmeric powder into warm water or milk.
- Add honey and stir well.
- Usage: Drink daily, preferably in the morning.

(e) Artichoke and Lemon Juice

Ingredients:

1 medium-sized artichoke

1 lemon

Instructions:

- Cook the artichoke until tender.
- Squeeze the lemon juice over the cooked artichoke.
- Usage: Eat as a side dish or snack.

(f) Beetroot and Apple Cider Vinegar Salad

Ingredients:

2 medium-sized beetroots

2 tablespoons of apple cider vinegar

1 tablespoon of olive oil

Instructions:

- Boil or roast the beetroots until tender.
- Slice the beetroots and mix with apple cider vinegar and olive oil.
- Usage: Serve as a salad.

(g) Turmeric Coconut Milk Smoothie

Ingredients:

1 cup of coconut milk

1 teaspoon of turmeric powder

1 banana (optional)

Honey (optional)

Instructions:

- Blend all ingredients until smooth.
- Usage: Drink as a snack or meal.

(h) Artichoke Garlic Roast

Ingredients:

2 medium-sized artichokes

2-3 garlic cloves

2 tablespoons of olive oil

Salt and pepper

Instructions:

- Clean and cut the artichokes into halves.
- Slice garlic cloves and place them inside the artichokes.
- Drizzle with olive oil and season with salt and pepper.
- Roast in the oven at 400°F (200°C) for 20-30 minutes.
- Usage: Serve as a side dish.

10.8 Gastritis: Herbs and Natural Remedies

1) Chamomile - Known for its soothing properties and can help with inflammation.
2) Licorice Root - Contains compounds that help protect the stomach lining.
3) Ginger - Helps with digestion and can reduce inflammation.
4) Peppermint - Calms the stomach and reduces nausea.
5) Slippery Elm - Forms a protective coating in the stomach and intestines.
6) Marshmallow Root - Has soothing properties and forms a protective layer.

7) Fennel - Relieves gas and bloating and helps with digestion.

8) Turmeric - Contains curcumin, which has anti-inflammatory properties.

9) Aloe Vera - Can soothe the stomach and help with healing.

10) Dandelion - Stimulates digestion and may help protect the stomach lining.

(a) Cabbage Juice

Ingredients:

1/2 cabbage (green or red)

2-3 stalks of celery

1 carrot

1 green apple

1 lemon

Instructions:

- Chop the cabbage and blend it with celery, carrot, green apple and lemon with some water until smooth.
- Strain the juice and discard the pulp.
- Drink half a cup of cabbage juice on an empty stomach daily.

(b) Cooling Peppermint Infusion

Ingredients:

1 tablespoon of dried peppermint leaves

1 cup of hot water

Instructions:

- Pour hot water over dried peppermint leaves.
- Let it steep for 5-10 minutes.
- Strain, chill and drink.

(c) Apple and Pear Compote

Ingredients:

2 apples, peeled and chopped

2 pears, peeled and chopped

1/4 cup of water

1 teaspoon of cinnamon

Instructions:

- Combine apples, pears, and water in a saucepan.
- Cook over medium heat until fruit is soft.
- Add cinnamon and stir.
- Serve warm or cold.
- Usage: Eat as a snack or dessert.

(d) Fennel and Carrot Soup

Ingredients:

1 cup of chopped fennel

1 cup of chopped carrots

4 cups of vegetable broth

1 tablespoon of olive oil

Salt and pepper to taste

Instructions:

- Sauté fennel and carrots in olive oil until softened.
- Add vegetable broth and bring to a boil.
- Simmer until vegetables are tender.
- Blend until smooth and season with salt and pepper.
- Usage: Serve as a meal or side dish.

(e) Slippery Elm Porridge

Ingredients:

1 tablespoon of slippery elm powder

1 cup of warm water or milk

Honey or sweetener (optional)

Instructions:

- Mix slippery elm powder with warm water or milk.
- Sweeten with honey if desired.
- Usage: Eat once daily, preferably on an empty stomach.

10.9 Herbs for Pancreas Health

1) Bitter Melon - Contains compounds that can help regulate blood sugar levels and support pancreatic function.
2) Licorice Root - Has anti-inflammatory properties and may protect the pancreas.
3) Milk Thistle - Contains silymarin, which may help protect the liver and pancreas.
4) Holy Basil - Known to improve pancreatic function and lower blood sugar levels.
5) Ginger - Contains anti-inflammatory compounds that can benefit the pancreas.
6) Turmeric - Contains curcumin, which has anti-inflammatory and antioxidant properties that can support pancreatic health.
7) Dandelion Root - Supports liver function and may benefit the pancreas as well.
8) Gymnema Sylvestre - Helps regulate blood sugar levels, which can support pancreatic health.
9) Aloe Vera - Contains compounds that may help regulate blood sugar and support the pancreas.
10) Cinnamon - Helps improve insulin sensitivity and supports pancreatic function.

10.9. Pancreatic Diseases: Herbs and Natural Remedies

(a) Grape Seed Extract Smoothie

Ingredients:

1 cup of low-fat yogurt or plant-based yogurt

1 cup of mixed berries

1 teaspoon of grape seed extract powder

Instructions:

- Blend all ingredients until smooth.
- Serve chilled.

(b) Bilberry Fruit Salad

Ingredients:

1 cup of bilberries or blueberries

1 apple, chopped

1 pear, chopped

1 tablespoon of lemon juice

Instructions:

- Mix all ingredients together in a bowl.
- Drizzle with lemon juice and toss.
- Usage: Enjoy as a snack or dessert.

(c) Goldenseal Herbal Tea

Ingredients:

1 teaspoon of dried goldenseal root

1 cup of water

Instructions:

- Boil 1 cup of water.
- Add dried goldenseal root.
- Let it steep for 10 minutes, then strain and drink.

(d) Olive Leaf Infusion

Ingredients:

1 tablespoon of dried olive leaves

1 cup of water

150

Instructions:

- Boil 1 cup of water.
- Add dried olive leaves.
- Let it steep for 10 minutes, then strain.

(e) Low-Fat Yogurt with Blueberries

Ingredients:

1 cup of low-fat yogurt or plant-based yogurt

1/2 cup of blueberries

1 teaspoon of honey (optional)

Instructions:

- Mix yogurt and blueberries together.
- Sweeten with honey if desired.

(f) Spinach and Kale Juice

Ingredients:

1 cup of fresh spinach

1 cup of fresh kale

1 apple

1 cup of water

Instructions:

- Blend all ingredients until smooth.
- Strain (if desired) and serve.

(g) Whole Grain Quinoa and Vegetables

Ingredients:

1 cup of cooked quinoa

1 cup of mixed vegetables (such as carrots, peas, and bell peppers)

1 tablespoon of olive oil

Salt and pepper to taste

Instructions:

- Sauté mixed vegetables in olive oil until tender.
- Add cooked quinoa and mix well.
- Season with salt and pepper.
- Usage: Serve as a meal or side dish.

(h) Pumpkin Soup with Ginger

Ingredients:

2 cups of pumpkin puree

1 tablespoon of grated ginger

2 cups of vegetable broth

1 tablespoon of olive oil

Salt and pepper to taste

Instructions:

- Sauté grated ginger in olive oil until fragrant.
- Add pumpkin puree and vegetable broth.
- Simmer for 10 minutes, then season with salt and pepper.
- Usage: Serve as a meal.

10.10. Respiratory Diseases: Herbs and Natural Remedies

1) Eucalyptus - Contains compounds that help clear congestion and improve respiratory function.
2) Peppermint - Contains menthol, which helps clear sinuses and alleviate respiratory discomfort.
3) Thyme - Has antibacterial and expectorant properties, useful for respiratory infections.
4) Mullein - Soothes the respiratory tract and helps clear congestion.
5) Licorice Root - Has anti-inflammatory properties and helps soothe the respiratory tract.

6) Oregano - Contains carvacrol, an antimicrobial compound that may benefit respiratory health.

7) Ginger - Helps reduce inflammation and soothe the respiratory system.

8) Elderberry - Has antiviral properties and may help alleviate respiratory symptoms.

9) Marshmallow Root - Soothes the throat and respiratory tract.

10) Lobelia - Acts as a bronchodilator and helps clear mucus.

(a) Eucalyptus Steam Inhalation

Ingredients:

A few drops of eucalyptus essential oil

A bowl of hot water

Instructions:

- Add a few drops of eucalyptus essential oil to a bowl of hot water.
- Lean over the bowl and cover your head with a towel to trap the steam.
- Inhale deeply for 5-10 minutes.
- Usage: Use as needed to relieve congestion.

(b) Licorice Root Tea

See natural recipes for Kidney and liver diseases.

(c) Thyme and Honey Syrup

Ingredients:

1 tablespoon of dried thyme

1 cup of water

1/2 cup of honey

Instructions:

- Boil water and add dried thyme.
- Let it steep for 10 minutes, then strain.
- Mix in honey until dissolved.

- Store in a glass jar.
- Usage: Take 1 tablespoon as needed.

(d) Ginger and Turmeric Tea

See natural recipes for Turmeric and Ginger Tea used for muscle health and pain relief.

(e) Mullein Leaf Decoction

Ingredients:

1 tablespoon of dried mullein leaves

1 cup of water

Instructions:

- Boil 1 cup of water.
- Add dried mullein leaves and simmer for 10 minutes.
- Strain and drink.

(f) Elderberry Syrup

Ingredients:

1 cup of dried elderberries

3 cups of water

1 cup of honey

Instructions:

- Boil dried elderberries in water until reduced by half.
- Strain and mix with honey until dissolved.
- Store in a glass jar.
- Usage: Take 1 tablespoon daily.

(f) Garlic and Honey Tonic

Ingredients:

1/2 cup of minced garlic

1 cup of honey

Instructions:

Mix minced garlic with honey.

Store in a glass jar for 1-2 days before use.

(g) Spicy Garlic Soup

Ingredients:

5 cloves of garlic, minced

1 onion, chopped

1 tablespoon of olive oil

4 cups of vegetable broth

1 teaspoon of cayenne pepper

Salt and pepper to taste

Instructions:

- Sauté garlic and onion in olive oil until softened.
- Add vegetable broth and cayenne pepper, and simmer for 20 minutes.
- Usage: Serve as a meal.

(h) Steamer Pot Herbal Blend for Inhalation

Ingredients:

1 teaspoon each of dried thyme, rosemary, and eucalyptus

2 cups of water

Instructions:

- Boil water and add the dried herbs.
- Lean over the pot and cover your head with a towel to trap the steam.
- Inhale deeply for 5-10 minutes.
- Usage: Use as needed to relieve congestion.

(i) Honey and Cinnamon Paste

Ingredients:

1 tablespoon of honey

1/2 teaspoon of cinnamon powder

Instructions:

- Mix honey and cinnamon until it turns into a paste.
- Usage: Take 1 tablespoon daily.

(j) Radish and Honey Syrup

Ingredients:

1 cup of grated radish

1/2 cup of honey

Instructions:

- Mix grated radish with honey.
- Let it sit for several hours until a syrup forms.
- Usage: Take 1 tablespoon daily.

(k) Peppermint Leaf Tea

See recipe under peppermint ginger tea for gastrointestinal diseases.

10.11. Seasonal Diseases (like Colds and Flu): Herbs and Natural Remedies

1) Elderberry - Contains compounds that can help boost the immune system and reduce the severity of cold and flu symptoms.
2) Echinacea - Often used to boost immunity and prevent or shorten the duration of colds and flu.
3) Ginger - Has anti-inflammatory properties and can help relieve symptoms like sore throat and congestion.
4) Garlic - Known for its antimicrobial properties, garlic can help boost the immune system.

5) Peppermint - Contains menthol, which can relieve nasal congestion and soothe a sore throat.

6) Thyme - Has antimicrobial properties and can help soothe coughs and sore throats.

7) Lemon Balm - Can help reduce symptoms of cold and flu, and is also calming.

8) Chamomile - Soothes the throat and helps with rest, which is important for recovery.

9) Licorice Root - Soothes the throat and has antiviral properties.

10) Rosemary - Contains compounds that may help reduce inflammation and boost immunity.

(a) Cinnamon and Clove Hot Drink

See Cinnamon and Clove Tea natural recipe used for diabetes.

(b) Nettle Leaf Infusion

See under natural recipes for kidney and liver diseases.

(c) Ginger Lemon Honey Tea

See under recipes for managing diabetes.

(d) Garlic and Honey Tonic

See under recipes support respiratory health.

(e) Thyme and Sage Herbal Steam

Ingredients:

1 tablespoon of dried thyme

1 tablespoon of dried sage

2 cups of boiling water

Instructions:
- Begin by placing the dried herbs in a spacious bowl.
- Pour boiling water over the herbs, covering them completely.
- Position yourself over the bowl, covering your head with a towel to trap the steam.
- Inhale the aromatic steam for 5 to 10 minutes, allowing the herbal vapors to soothe and refresh.

(f) Chamomile and Lemon Balm Tea

Ingredients:

1 teaspoon of dried chamomile flowers

1 teaspoon of dried lemon balm leaves

1 cup of hot water

Instructions:

- Pour hot water over the dried herbs.
- Let it steep for 5-10 minutes.
- Strain and drink.

(g) Echinacea Herbal Tea

Ingredients:

1 teaspoon of dried echinacea root or leaves

1 cup of hot water

Instructions:

- Place dried echinacea in a heatproof container.
- Pour hot water over the dried echinacea.
- Allow it to steep for 5-10 minutes.
- Strain the infusion and enjoy.

(h) Ginger Turmeric Immunity Boosting Smoothie

Ingredients:

1-inch piece of fresh ginger

1 teaspoon of turmeric powder

1 cup of orange juice

1 cup of frozen mixed berries

Instructions:

- Blend all ingredients until smooth.
- Serve chilled.

(i) Oregano Oil Steam Inhalation

Ingredients:

A few drops of oregano essential oil

A bowl of hot water

Instructions:

- Boil water until it reaches a rolling boil.
- Pour the boiling water into a bowl or basin.
- Add a few drops of oregano oil to the hot water.
- Position yourself over the bowl, covering your head with a towel to create a steam tent.
- Inhale the steam for 5-10 minutes to reap its therapeutic benefits.

(j) Cayenne Pepper Lemonade

Ingredients:

1 tablespoon of fresh lemon juice

1 teaspoon of cayenne pepper

1 tablespoon of honey

1 cup of warm water

Instructions:

- Mix all ingredients together until honey is dissolved.
- Garnish with lemon slices and mint leaves if desired.

(k) Apple Cider Vinegar Immune Tonic

Ingredients:

1 tablespoon of apple cider vinegar

1 tablespoon of honey

1 cup of warm water

Instructions:

- Mix all ingredients together until honey is dissolved.
- Usage: Drink once daily.

10.12 Hormonal Issues: Herbs and Natural Remedies

1) Flaxseeds: Flaxseeds are a potent source of ALA (alpha-linolenic acid), a type of plant-derived omega-3 fatty acid. Additionally, they contain lignans, which are phytoestrogens, mimicking estrogen's action in the body. Compared to other plant foods, flaxseeds boast up to 800 times more lignans. Typically found in ground or oil form, they make excellent additions to salads as dressings or can be blended into smoothies.

2) Chaste Tree Berry (Vitex Agnus-Castus): Primarily beneficial for women's health, chaste tree berry is renowned for its role in regulating menstrual cycles, alleviating premenstrual syndrome (PMS) symptoms, and managing menopausal discomfort. It's commonly consumed as a capsule, tincture, or tea.

3) Maca Root: Maca root is celebrated for its capacity to boost energy, enhance stamina, and invigorate libido. It's also valued for its ability to rebalance estrogen levels and alleviate menopausal symptoms. Often available in powder form, it can be seamlessly incorporated into smoothies, oatmeal, or baked goods.

4) Black Cohosh: Frequently utilized to alleviate menopausal symptoms such as hot flashes, night sweats, and menstrual pain, black cohosh is typically ingested in capsule or tincture form.

5) Ashwagandha: Functioning as an adaptogenic herb, ashwagandha aids the body in combating various stressors, whether physical, chemical, or biological. It's reputed for its potential to enhance thyroid function, support adrenal health, and mitigate anxiety and stress. Available in capsules, powders, or liquid extracts, ashwagandha offers versatile consumption options.

6) Red Raspberry Leaf: Recognized for its advantages during pregnancy, red raspberry leaf also proves beneficial for alleviating menstrual cramps and heavy bleeding during menstruation. It's commonly enjoyed as a soothing tea.

7) Dong Quai: Dubbed the "female ginseng," Dong Quai finds application in relieving menstrual discomfort, regulating irregular menstrual cycles, and alleviating menopausal symptoms. It can be found in capsules, tinctures, and is frequently featured in herbal teas.Licorice Root

8) Licorice root can affect estrogen and progesterone levels, making it useful for various hormonal issues, including fertility and menstrual irregularities. It's also used for adrenal support. Can be taken as capsules, teas, or chewed as a stick.

(a) Flaxseed Smoothie

Ingredients:

1 tablespoon of ground flaxseed

1 cup of mixed berries (blueberries, strawberries, raspberries, etc.)

1 handful of spinach

1 cup of almond milk

1 scoop of protein powder (optional)

1 teaspoon of honey or sweetener (optional)

Instructions:

- Combine all the ingredients in a blender.
- Blend until a smooth consistency is achieved.
- Sample the mixture and adjust sweetness to your preference, if needed.
- Chill the mixture before serving.

(b) Salmon Salad

Ingredients:

Grilled salmon

Leafy greens

Avocado

Olive oil

Instructions:

- Grill the salmon fillets.
- Combine grilled salmon with leafy greens and avocado.
- Drizzle with olive oil and serve.

(c) Tofu Stir-Fry

Ingredients:

Tofu

Bell peppers

Broccoli

Carrots

Ginger

Garlic

Stir-fry sauce

Salt and pepper to taste

Instructions:

- Sauté tofu with colorful vegetables like bell peppers, broccoli, and carrots in a ginger-garlic sauce. Add soya sauce for taste.
- Serve with rice or noodles.

(d) Quinoa Breakfast Bowl

Ingredients:

Cooked quinoa

Greek yogurt

Mixed berries

Almonds

Honey

Instructions:

- Cook quinoa.
- Top with Greek yogurt, mixed berries, almonds, and a drizzle of honey.

(e) Herbal Infusion

Ingredients:

Red clover

Dong quai

Licorice root

Instructions:

- Brew a blend of hormone-balancing herbs in hot water.
- Strain and enjoy as a tea.

(f) Sweet Potato and Kale Hash

Ingredients:

Sweet potatoes

Kale

Onions

Garlic

Olive oil

Instructions:

- Sauté diced sweet potatoes and kale with onions and garlic in olive oil.
- Serve as a side or main dish.

(g) Turmeric and Ginger Stir-Fry (with tofu, vegetable of your choice and chicken)

Ingredients:

Tofu or chicken

Turmeric

Ginger

Garlic

Bell peppers

Broccoli

Snap peas

Salt and pepper to taste

Instructions:
- Cook sliced tofu or chicken with turmeric, ginger, garlic, and vegetables.
- Serve with rice or noodles.

(h) Berry Overnight Oats

Ingredients:
Rolled oats
Almond milk
Greek yogurt
Chia seeds
Mixed berries

Instructions:
- Mix rolled oats with almond milk, Greek yogurt, chia seeds, and berries.
- Refrigerate overnight and have it for breakfast next morning or as a snack.

(i) Lentil Soup

Ingredients:
Lentils
Diced tomatoes
Carrots
Celery
Onions
Thyme
Oregano
Salt and pepper to taste

Instructions:
- Soak lentils for 6 hours.
- Simmer lentils with diced vegetables and herbs for a hearty soup.

(j) Green Smoothie Bowl

Ingredients:

Spinach

Kale

Banana

Avocado

Almond milk

Protein powder

Instructions:

- Blend spinach, kale, banana, avocado, almond milk, and protein powder until smooth.
- Top with nuts, seeds, and fresh fruit.

(k) Sesame Ginger Salmon

Ingredients:

Salmon fillets

Soy sauce

Sesame oil

Ginger

Garlic

Instructions:

- Marinate salmon in soy sauce, sesame oil, ginger, and garlic.
- Cook the salmon by baking or grilling for approximately 12-15 minutes, or until it easily flakes apart when tested with a fork.

(l) Avocado Chocolate Mousse

Ingredients:

Ripe avocado

Cocoa powder

Honey or maple syrup

Almond milk

Instructions:
- Blend ripe avocado with cocoa powder, honey, and almond milk until smooth.
- Chill and serve.

(m) Cauliflower Rice Stir-Fry

Ingredients:
Cauliflower rice
Mixed vegetables
Tofu or chicken
Stir-fry sauce

Instructions:
- Sauté cauliflower rice with mixed vegetables and protein.
- Add a homemade stir-fry sauce for flavor.

10.13 Metabolic Diseases and Weight Control: Herbs and Natural Remedies

1) Green Tea - Rich in antioxidants called catechins, particularly epigallocatechin gallate (EGCG), green tea is known to boost metabolism and aid in fat burning. Its caffeine content further enhances these effects. Regular consumption of green tea not only supports weight management but also contributes to improved cardiovascular health.

2) Cinnamon - Cinnamon is recognized for its ability to enhance insulin sensitivity, making it valuable for regulating blood sugar levels, especially in individuals with metabolic conditions like type 2 diabetes. By improving insulin sensitivity, cinnamon facilitates more efficient glucose utilization, reducing fat accumulation and assisting in weight control. Additionally, its flavorful profile can enhance dishes without the need for added sugars, helping to reduce cravings.

3) Ginger - Ginger possesses thermogenic properties, which means it can increase the body's heat production and, in turn, enhance metabolism. This property, along with its potential to regulate blood sugar levels and reduce appetite, makes ginger a useful herb for weight

management. Additionally, ginger has anti-inflammatory properties that can improve overall health and contribute to metabolic wellness.

4) Fenugreek - Fenugreek seeds contain a type of soluble fiber that slows down digestion and the absorption of carbohydrates. This can lead to improved blood sugar control and reduced appetite, both of which are crucial for weight management. Fenugreek has also been studied for its potential to increase insulin sensitivity, further supporting metabolic health.

5) Garcinia Cambogia - Garcinia cambogia is a fruit known for its rind, which contains hydroxycitric acid (HCA). This compound has garnered interest due to its potential to inhibit the enzyme ATP-citrate lyase, which is implicated in fat storage. Additionally, it's believed to influence appetite by boosting serotonin levels. Despite some studies indicating modest weight loss benefits, further research is required to validate the effectiveness and safety of Garcinia cambogia.

6) Ginseng - Ginseng, an adaptogenic herb, aids the body in adapting to stressors and enhancing overall resilience. Studies have indicated its role in regulating blood sugar levels, boosting insulin sensitivity, and elevating energy expenditure, factors that support weight management efforts. Moreover, ginseng's potential benefits extend to metabolic health, encompassing improved immune function and diminished inflammation.

7) Bitter Orange - Bitter orange contains synephrine, a compound that may increase metabolism and promote fat burning. However, it can have side effects and interact with certain medications, particularly those affecting the cardiovascular system. Despite its potential, caution is advised when using bitter orange for weight management, especially for individuals with existing health conditions.

8) Dandelion - Dandelion root tea acts as a natural diuretic, which can help reduce water weight and bloating. Beyond its diuretic properties, dandelion supports liver function and aids digestion, which can indirectly support weight management. The herb is also rich in vitamins and minerals, contributing to overall health.

9) Turmeric - Curcumin, found in turmeric, possesses potent antioxidant and anti-inflammatory abilities. It can help alleviate inflammation linked to obesity and metabolic disorders. Additionally, curcumin could enhance insulin sensitivity and promote weight loss by boosting metabolic function.

10) Licorice Root - Licorice root has been shown to regulate blood sugar levels and reduce cravings for sweets, which can be beneficial for weight management. However, it should be used with caution, as it can increase blood pressure in some individuals. It's essential to monitor

consumption and consult a healthcare provider if considering licorice root for metabolic health or weight control.

(a) Turmeric Roasted Vegetables

Ingredients:
Mixed vegetables (carrots, bell peppers, broccoli, cauliflower) – 4 cups
Olive oil – 2 tbsp
Turmeric powder – 1 tsp
Garlic powder – 1/2 tsp
Salt and pepper to taste

Instructions:
- Heat the oven to 400°F (200°C).
- Combine vegetables with olive oil, turmeric, garlic powder, salt, and pepper in a large bowl, making sure they are well-coated.
- Arrange the vegetables in a single layer on a baking sheet.
- Roast in the oven for 25-30 minutes, stirring once at the midway point, until the vegetables are tender and have a golden color.

(b) Quinoa Salad with Chickpeas and Spinach

Ingredients:
Cooked quinoa – 2 cups
Canned chickpeas, rinsed and drained – 1 cup
Fresh spinach, chopped – 2 cups
Cherry tomatoes, halved – 1 cup
Red onion, finely chopped – 1/4 cup
Lemon juice – 2 tbsp
Olive oil – 1 tbsp
Salt and pepper to taste

Instructions:
- In a large bowl, combine the quinoa, chickpeas, spinach, cherry tomatoes, and red onion.

- In a smaller bowl, thoroughly mix lemon juice, olive oil, salt, and pepper by whisking vigorously.
- Pour the dressing over the salad and toss gently to ensure it is evenly distributed.
- Serve immediately or store in the refrigerator until needed.

(c) Baked Salmon with Dill and Lemon

Ingredients:

Salmon fillets – 4 (6 oz each)

Fresh dill, chopped – 2 tbsp

Lemon, thinly sliced – 1

Olive oil – 2 tbsp

Salt and pepper to taste

Instructions:

- Heat the oven to 375°F (190°C).
- Place salmon fillets on a baking sheet lined with parchment paper.
- Drizzle the fillets with olive oil and season well with salt and pepper.
- Top each fillet with slices of lemon and a dash of dill.
- Cook in the oven for 15-20 minutes, or until the salmon is fully cooked and flakes easily with a fork.

(d) Ginger-Lemon Chicken Stir-Fry

Ingredients:

Chicken breast, thinly sliced – 1 lb (450 g)

Fresh ginger, minced – 1 tbsp

Garlic, minced – 2 cloves

Bell pepper, sliced – 1

Snow peas – 1 cup

Soy sauce – 2 tbsp

Lemon juice – 1 tbsp

Olive or sesame oil – 1 tbsp

Salt and pepper to taste

Instructions:

- Heat oil in a large skillet or wok over medium-high heat.
- Sauté ginger and garlic in the heated oil for about 30 seconds until their fragrance blooms.
- Introduce the chicken into the skillet, stirring and frying until it begins to brown.
- Toss in the bell pepper and snow peas, cooking until the veggies reach a tender-crisp texture.
- Blend in soy sauce and lemon juice, and season with salt and pepper.
- Continue cooking for another minute until all ingredients meld together seamlessly and the chicken is fully cooked.
- Serve the dish piping hot.

(e) Chia Seed Pudding

Ingredients:

Chia seeds – 1/4 cup

Almond milk (or any other plant-based milk) – 1 cup

Maple syrup or honey – 1 tbsp (optional)

Vanilla extract – 1/2 tsp

Instructions:

- In a bowl, mix the chia seeds, almond milk, maple syrup (if using), and vanilla extract.
- Stir well to combine, then let sit for 5 minutes.
- Stir again to break up any clumps and refrigerate for at least 2 hours or overnight.
- The pudding should be thick and creamy.
- Serve chilled, topped with fresh fruit or nuts if desired.

10.14 Headache: Herbs and Natural Remedies

1) **Peppermint** - Peppermint contains menthol, which can relax muscles and ease pain. It's often used in topical applications to relieve tension headaches. Drinking peppermint tea or applying peppermint oil to the temples can be effective.

2) **Ginger** - Its anti-inflammatory properties help alleviate headaches, especially migraines. Consuming ginger tea or incorporating ginger into meals can be beneficial.

3) **Lavender** - Lavender is known for its calming properties. Inhaling lavender essential oil or applying it topically can help reduce headache symptoms. Lavender tea can also provide soothing relief.

4) **Feverfew** - Feverfew has been traditionally used to prevent migraines. It contains parthenolide, a compound that can reduce inflammation and blood vessel constriction. It's commonly taken in capsule form or used to make tea.

5) **Chamomile** - Chamomile has relaxing and anti-inflammatory properties. Drinking chamomile tea can help soothe headaches and promote relaxation.

(a) Peppermint Tea

Ingredients:

Fresh peppermint leaves – 1 handful (or 1 peppermint tea bag)

Hot water – 1 cup

Honey or lemon (optional)

Instructions:

- Place the peppermint leaves or tea bag in a cup.
- Pour hot water over the leaves or bag.
- Let it steep for 5-10 minutes.
- Strain (if using fresh leaves) and enjoy, optionally sweetened with honey or a squeeze of lemon.

(b) Ginger Lemon Honey Tea

See under recipes for managing diabetes.

(c) Lavender and Chamomile Tea

Ingredients:

Dried lavender – 1 tsp

Dried chamomile flowers – 1 tsp

Hot water – 1 cup

Honey (optional)

Instructions:

- Combine the lavender and chamomile in a cup.
- Pour hot water over the herbs.
- Let steep for 5-10 minutes.
- Strain and enjoy, optionally sweetened with honey.

(d) Feverfew Tea

Ingredients:

Fresh or dried feverfew leaves – 1 tsp

Hot water – 1 cup

Honey (optional)

Instructions:

- Set the feverfew leaves in a cup.
- Pour hot water over the leaves.
- Allow the mixture to steep for 5-10 minutes.
- Strain the infusion and savor, optionally adding honey for sweetness

CHAPTER 11: HOW TO GROW YOUR OWN MEDICINAL HERBS AT HOME

11.1 Choosing Medicinal Herbs to Grow

Growing medicinal herbs at home is a rewarding endeavor, allowing individuals to access natural remedies while cultivating a closer relationship with nature. However, choosing the right medicinal herbs to grow requires careful consideration of several factors, including understanding their growing conditions and care requirements.

Medicinal herbs vary widely in their preferences for soil type, sunlight, water, and climate. Understanding these requirements is crucial for successful cultivation. Each herb has unique needs, and providing the right environment is key to maximizing their therapeutic properties. Moreover, some herbs are perennial, while others are annual or biennial, influencing how long they can be harvested. Proper knowledge can help us to avoid common pitfalls, such as planting shade-loving herbs in direct sunlight or neglecting the water needs of moisture-loving plants.

Factors to Consider When Selecting Medicinal Herbs

Selecting medicinal herbs involves considering personal health needs, space availability, climate, and growing conditions.

- *Personal Health Needs*: One should first identify the health issues they want to address with medicinal herbs. For example, those prone to colds might benefit from growing echinacea, while people seeking relaxation might prefer lavender. Choosing herbs based on specific health goals ensures a personalized approach to wellness.
- *Space Availability*: The space available for gardening plays a significant role in herb selection. Small spaces like windowsills or balconies might be suitable for herbs that thrive in pots, such as mint or cilantro. Larger spaces, such as gardens, offer the flexibility to grow a wider range of herbs, including those that spread out or grow tall.
- *Climate*: Local climate conditions are crucial when choosing herbs to grow. Some herbs, like rosemary, prefer warm, dry climates, while others, like mint, thrive in cooler, moist environments. Understanding the climate's influence helps in selecting herbs that will flourish naturally, minimizing the need for extensive modifications or protections.
- *Growing Conditions*: Each herb has specific preferences for soil type, sunlight, and water. You should evaluate their available resources and choose herbs that align with their conditions. For

example, Mediterranean herbs like oregano and sage prefer well-drained soil and full sun, while marsh-loving herbs like valerian require moist, shaded environments.

Medicinal Herbs Suitable for Home Cultivation

Various medicinal herbs are well-suited for home cultivation, each offering unique therapeutic properties and uses. These herbs can be categorized based on their applications.

- *Herbs for Immune Support*: Echinacea and elderberry are popular for boosting immunity. Echinacea is a perennial herb that thrives in well-drained soil and full sun. Elderberry, a deciduous shrub, prefers similar conditions and produces berries rich in antioxidants.

- *Herbs for Heart Health*: Growing heart-healthy herbs like basil and fennel is rewarding. Basil, rich in antioxidants, thrives in sunny, warm spots and requires well-drained soil. Fennel, packed with fiber and potassium, also needs a sunny location, and prefers well-drained soil. Both herbs support cardiovascular wellness. Basil is easy to propagate, while fennel grows well from seeds sown outdoors in mid-spring. Regular watering and harvesting enhance their growth.

- *Herbs for Relaxation and Sleep*: Lavender and chamomile are excellent choices for relaxation. Lavender, a hardy perennial, enjoys full sun and well-drained soil, while chamomile, an annual herb, prefers moderate sunlight and well-drained soil. Both herbs can be used to make calming teas or essential oils.

- *Herbs for Digestion*: Peppermint, ginger, and cilantro are commonly used to aid digestion. Peppermint is a hardy perennial that thrives in partial shade and moist soil. Ginger, a tropical plant, requires warm temperatures and moist, well-drained soil. Cilantro is an annual herb that grows best in cool weather with moderate sunlight. These herbs can be used fresh or dried to make soothing teas or added to dishes.

- *Herbs for Skin Care*: Aloe vera, calendula, and parsley are known for their skin-healing properties. Aloe vera is a succulent that thrives in dry, sunny conditions, while calendula, an annual, prefers moderate sunlight and well-drained soil. Parsley is a biennial herb that grows best in full sun and moist, well-drained soil. All three herbs can be used to create soothing topical treatments.

11.2 Setting Up Your Herb Garden

Selecting the Right Location

-   Choosing the ideal location for an herb garden involves careful consideration of several key factors. The primary factor is sunlight exposure. Most herbs thrive in full sun, which means they require at least six to eight hours of direct sunlight daily. When selecting a location, it's important to observe how the sunlight moves across the garden throughout the day to ensure optimal exposure for the herbs.

-   Soil quality is another vital aspect. Herbs typically prefer well-drained soil with a rich, loamy texture. Before planting, it's crucial to evaluate the soil quality in the selected area. If the soil is poor or compacted, it may need improvement through organic matter or other soil amendments.

-   Drainage is also critical for an herb garden. Herbs generally do not fare well in waterlogged conditions, so it's important to choose a location where water does not accumulate after rain. If the garden area tends to retain water, it may be necessary to install drainage systems or consider alternative gardening methods like raised beds or containers.

-   Accessibility should also be factored in when selecting the garden's location. The herb garden should be easily accessible for maintenance and harvesting. Positioning the garden near the kitchen or a frequently used pathway ensures convenience. Additionally, accessibility facilitates regular care, such as watering and pruning, which is essential for healthy herb growth.

11.3 Different Gardening Methods

Several gardening methods are suitable for growing medicinal herbs at home, each offering unique benefits.

-   Raised beds are a popular choice, which provides excellent drainage and allows you to control soil quality. Raised beds are ideal for areas with poor soil conditions or where space is limited. They can be constructed from various materials, including wood, stone, or recycled materials, and offer the added benefit of easier access, reducing the need for bending over.

- Containers are another flexible option for herb gardening. Growing herbs in containers allows for mobility, enabling the movement of plants to optimal locations based on seasonal changes or sunlight availability. Containers also offer control over soil conditions, making them suitable for herbs with specific requirements. It's important to select containers with adequate drainage holes to prevent waterlogging.

- Vertical gardens provide a space-saving solution for herb cultivation. Using structures such as trellises, wall-mounted planters, or stacked containers, vertical gardens maximize space by growing herbs upward. This method is particularly useful for small spaces or urban environments where ground space is limited.

- Indoor herb gardens cater to those without outdoor space or in regions with challenging climates. Growing herbs indoors requires proper planning for light and space. Using grow lights or placing herbs near sunny windows ensures they receive sufficient light. Indoor herb gardens offer the advantage of year-round cultivation, allowing for fresh herbs even in winter.

11.4. Preparing the Soil

Proper soil preparation is crucial for successful herb gardening. Soil testing is the first step, as it helps identify the soil's pH level and nutrient composition. Testing kits are available for home use, or samples can be sent to local agricultural extension offices for analysis. Knowing the soil's characteristics allows for targeted amendments to address deficiencies or imbalances.

- Enriching the soil with organic materials is advantageous for cultivating most herbs. By adding compost or decayed manure, you enhance the soil's fertility, texture, and microbial activity, which all support robust herb growth. It's beneficial to mix organic substances into the soil prior to planting to create a nourishing environment for the herbs.

- It is also crucial to keep the soil pH within an ideal range for herb growth. Herbs generally thrive in a slightly acidic to neutral pH, usually between 6.0 and 7.5. An imbalance in soil pH, either too high or too low, can obstruct the absorption of nutrients and adversely affect the health of the herbs. Adjustments to the soil pH can be made using lime or sulfur according to the findings from soil tests.

- In addition to soil amendments, it's important to monitor and adjust the soil's moisture retention. Herbs generally prefer well-drained soil, so adding materials like sand or perlite can improve drainage if the soil is too heavy or clayey. Conversely, if the soil is too sandy and doesn't retain moisture, incorporating organic matter can help enhance water-holding capacity.

By following these guidelines, you can create an optimal environment for your herb gardens, ensuring healthy, robust growth and a bountiful harvest.

11.5 Propagation and Planting Medicinal Herbs

Growing medicinal herbs provides the satisfaction of cultivating personal health remedies, and propagating them is an essential skill. There are various methods of propagation, each with its own set of advantages. Once propagated, these herbs can be successfully planted in gardens or containers, with proper attention to spacing, planting depth, and watering techniques.

Overview of Propagation Methods

Medicinal herbs can be propagated through several methods, including seeds, cuttings, divisions, and transplanting. Each method has unique benefits and challenges, so understanding these techniques helps in choosing the best approach for one's needs.

- Seeds: Propagating herbs from seeds is economical and offers a wide variety of options. Many herbs, such as basil, parsley, and dill, grow well from seeds. Starting herbs from seeds requires patience, as germination can take time, and seedlings need careful nurturing. However, it provides the flexibility to select specific varieties and is ideal for those who enjoy the process of nurturing plants from their earliest stages.
- Cuttings: Using cuttings is an efficient way to propagate woody or semi-woody herbs like rosemary, thyme, and mint. Cuttings are portions of stems or branches taken from a parent plant and rooted to create new plants. This method allows you to replicate desired plant traits. Cuttings root best when taken from healthy, mature plants, and they typically require a rooting medium and consistent moisture.
- Divisions: Division involves separating mature herb plants into smaller sections, each with its own roots and shoots. This method is suitable for herbs that spread through underground rhizomes or form clumps, such as lemon balm and chives. Division is best done during the

dormant season or early spring when the plant is not actively growing. It helps rejuvenate overgrown herbs and encourages vigorous new growth.

- Transplanting: Transplanting involves moving herb seedlings or young plants from one location to another, usually from indoor pots to an outdoor garden. This method is ideal for herbs started indoors or purchased as young plants. Transplanting allows you to control early growing conditions before placing herbs in their final location. Careful handling during transplanting is crucial to avoid damaging roots.

Step-by-Step Instructions for Planting

After propagating medicinal herbs, the next step is planting them in the garden or containers. Proper planting techniques ensure healthy growth and a bountiful harvest.

- Spacing: Adequate spacing is vital for herb health, as it allows air circulation and prevents overcrowding. The spacing requirements vary by herb type. For example, larger herbs like rosemary may need 18 to 24 inches of space, while smaller herbs like thyme can be planted closer together. Overcrowding can lead to competition for resources and increased susceptibility to diseases.
- Planting Depth: The planting depth is critical for establishing healthy herbs. Generally, seeds should be planted at a depth of two to three times their diameter, while seedlings should be planted at the same depth as they were in their previous containers. For cuttings and divisions, the planting depth should cover the roots without burying the stem or leaves. Planting too deeply can cause stem rot, while planting too shallowly can expose roots to drying out.
- Watering Techniques: Proper watering is essential for newly planted herbs. After planting, the soil should be thoroughly watered to settle the roots. Consistent moisture is vital during the initial growth stages, but overwatering should be avoided. Herbs generally prefer well-drained soil, so it's important to monitor soil moisture and adjust watering based on weather conditions. Mulching around the plants can help retain soil moisture and regulate temperature.
- Container Planting: Planting herbs in containers offers flexibility and is ideal for small spaces or indoor gardening. When planting in containers, ensure that each pot has drainage holes to prevent waterlogging. Use a well-draining potting mix and select containers that are appropriately sized for the herb's mature size. As with garden planting, maintain consistent moisture and avoid letting the soil dry out completely.

11.6 Herb Care and Maintenance

Maintaining healthy medicinal herbs requires ongoing care and attention to ensure they thrive and offer their beneficial properties. Key aspects of herb care include watering, fertilizing, pruning, and pest control, all of which contribute to robust plant growth. Additionally, understanding how to identify and manage common pests and diseases, as well as the proper techniques for harvesting herbs for optimal potency, helps maintain a thriving herb garden.

Essential Care Tasks

- Watering: Consistent watering is crucial for healthy herb growth. Most herbs prefer well-drained soil and do not tolerate waterlogged conditions. It's important to water herbs deeply and allow the soil to dry slightly between waterings to prevent root rot. However, some herbs, like mint, prefer consistently moist soil, so understanding the specific needs of each herb is key to effective watering.

- Fertilizing: Herbs generally benefit from light fertilization, as excessive feeding can lead to rapid, leggy growth that diminishes flavor and medicinal potency. Using organic fertilizers, such as compost or well-rotted manure, enriches the soil without overwhelming the herbs. It's typically best to apply fertilizer at the beginning of the growing season and again after a significant harvest to support continued growth.

- Pruning: Regular pruning encourages bushy growth and prevents herbs from becoming too woody or leggy. Pruning also helps manage the size and shape of herbs, which is particularly useful for container gardens or small spaces. Pruning should focus on removing dead or damaged leaves and stems, as well as harvesting fresh growth to stimulate new development.

- Pest Control: Pests can significantly impact herb health, so it's important to monitor plants regularly and address infestations promptly. Using natural pest control methods, such as neem oil or insecticidal soap, helps protect herbs without introducing harmful chemicals. Encouraging beneficial insects, like ladybugs, which prey on common herb pests, is also effective.

Identifying Pests and Diseases

Medicinal herbs are susceptible to various pests and diseases, but early identification and natural management strategies can mitigate damage.

179

- Common Pests: Aphids, spider mites, and whiteflies are common pests that affect medicinal herbs. These insects suck sap from plants, leading to stunted growth or distorted leaves. Handpicking or spraying with a strong jet of water can dislodge these pests. For severe infestations, applying neem oil or insecticidal soap can help control populations.
- Common Diseases: Fungal diseases, such as powdery mildew and downy mildew, often affect herbs in humid conditions. These diseases cause a white, powdery coating or fuzzy spots on leaves, leading to weakened plants. Improving air circulation, avoiding overhead watering, and applying fungicidal sprays can help manage these diseases. Proper spacing and pruning also reduce the risk of fungal infections.

Harvesting Herbs for Optimal Potency

Harvesting herbs correctly ensures maximum medicinal potency and flavor.

- Best Time of Day: The optimal time of day to harvest herbs is in the morning, after the dew has dried but before the day's heat. This timing preserves essential oils and keeps the herbs fresh.
- Harvesting Techniques: When harvesting, it's important to use clean, sharp scissors or pruning shears to avoid damaging the plant. For leafy herbs, harvesting from the top encourages bushy growth. For herbs with flowers, like chamomile, cutting the blossoms regularly stimulates more blooms. Always leave enough foliage for the plant to continue growing.
- Post-Harvest Handling: After harvesting, it's crucial to handle herbs properly to retain their potency. Drying herbs is a common method for preserving them. Herbs can be air-dried by hanging them in a cool, dark, well-ventilated space or dried using a dehydrator. Alternatively, fresh herbs can be stored in the refrigerator or frozen for later use. Proper storage prevents degradation and maintains the herbs' medicinal properties.

By focusing on essential care tasks, identifying, and managing pests and diseases, and employing effective harvesting techniques, you can maintain healthy, vibrant medicinal herbs that provide valuable health benefits.

EXTRA CONTENT

Uncover a treasure trove of extra content and additional resources waiting for you to explore and enjoy.

As a personal gift from the author, you will have access to exclusive bonuses such as:

- **Complete video lessons by Barbara O'Neill** (Healing the Gut, How to Fight Chronic Fatigue, How to Improve Your Mental Health, and more)
- **Herbal Topical Remedies**: Crafting Salves, Balms, Creams, and Ointments for Natural Healing

Scan the QR code or follow the link below to access everything:

https://www.boundlesspublishingpress.com/herbal-medicine-paperback-extra

----

A MESSAGE FROM THE AUTHOR:

As the author of this book, I have dedicated countless hours and a great deal of passion to its creation, aiming to provide readers with valuable insights and genuine inspiration. I truly hope that it resonates with you and enriches your understanding or appreciation of the topic. If you find this book impactful, I kindly ask that you consider leaving a review on Amazon. Your feedback is not only tremendously appreciated, but it is also crucial in helping to enhance the visibility of this work to other potential readers.

Scan the QR code or follow the link below for more information:

https://www.boundlesspublishingpress.com/feedback

REFERENCES

Capasso, F., Gaginella, T., Grandolini, G., & Izzo, A. (2003). The complexity of herbal medicines. *Phytotherapy,* Springer.

Chatfield, K., Salehi, B., Sharifi-Rad, J., & Afshar, L. (2018). Applying an ethical framework to herbal medicine. *Evidence-based Complementary and Alternative Medicine: eCAM, 2018.*

Dresler, M., & Repantis, D. (2015). Cognitive enhancement in humans. In S. Knafo & C. Venero (Eds.), *Cognitive Enhancement: Pharmacologic, Environmental and Genetic Factors* (pp. 273–306). Elsevier, Amsterdam.

El-Dahiyat, F., Rashrash, M., Abuhamdah, S., Abu Farha, R., & Babar, Z.-U.-D. (2020). Herbal medicines: A cross-sectional study to evaluate the prevalence and predictors of use among Jordanian adults. *Journal of Pharmaceutical Policy and Practice, 13*(2). https://doi.org/10.1186/s40545-019-0200-3

Fan, M., Zhang, X., Song, H., & Zhang, Y. (2023). Dandelion (Taraxacum Genus): A review of chemical constituents and pharmacological effects. *Molecules (Basel, Switzerland), 28*(13), 5022. https://doi.org/10.3390/molecules28135022

Firenzuoli, F., & Gori, L. (2007). Herbal medicine today: Clinical and research issues. *Evidence-Based Complementary and Alternative Medicine, 4,* 37-40. https://doi.org/10.1093/ecam/nem096

Fung, F. Y., & Linn, Y. C. (2015). Developing traditional Chinese medicine in the era of evidence-based medicine: Current evidence and challenges. *Evidence-Based Complementary and Alternative Medicine: eCAM, 2015,* 425037. https://doi.org/10.1155/2015/425037

Fung, F. Y., & Linn, Y. C. (2015). Developing traditional Chinese medicine in the era of evidence-based medicine: Current evidences and challenges. *Evidence-Based Complementary and Alternative Medicine: eCAM, 2015,* 425037. https://doi.org/10.1155/2015/425037

Goldman, P. (2001). Herbal medicines today and the roots of modern pharmacology. *Annals of Internal Medicine, 135*(8), 594-600.

Liu, Z. (2010). Basic principles of CM herbal formulation. In *Essentials of Chinese Medicine*. Liu, Z. (ed.). London, Springer.

Mamtani, R., Cheema, S., MacRae, B., Alrouh, H., Lopez, T., ElHajj, M., & Mahfoud, Z. (2015). Herbal and nutritional supplement use among college students in Qatar. *Eastern Mediterranean Health Journal, 21,* 39.

Matole, V., Thorat, Y., Ghurghure, S. M., Ingle, S., Birajdar, A., Nangare, G., Safwan, M., Madur, S., Patil, S., Bagalkote, Z. A., & Sakhare, A. (2021). A brief review on herbal medicines. *Research Journal of Pharmacognosy and Phytochemistry.*

Mehl-Madrona, L. (2003). Native American medicine: Herbal pharmacology, therapies, and elder care. In H. Selin (Ed.), *Medicine across cultures: Science across cultures: The history of non-Western science* (Vol. 3). Springer, Dordrecht. https://doi.org/10.1007/0-306-48094-8_11

Mehl-Madrona, L. (2003). Native American medicine: Herbal pharmacology, therapies, and elder care. In H. Selin (Ed.), *Medicine across cultures: Science across cultures: The history of non-Western science* (Vol. 3). Springer, Dordrecht. https://doi.org/10.1007/0-306-48094-8_11

Mocanu, M. L., & Amariei, S. (2022). Elderberries-A source of bioactive compounds with antiviral action. *Plants (Basel, Switzerland), 11*(6), 740. https://doi.org/10.3390/plants11060740

Mocanu, M. L., & Amariei, S. (2022). Elderberries-A source of bioactive compounds with antiviral action. *Plants (Basel, Switzerland), 11*(6), 740. https://doi.org/10.3390/plants11060740

Msomi, N. Z., & Simelane, M. B. C. (2018). Herbal medicine. In P. F. Builders (Ed.), *IntechOpen*. https://doi.org/10.5772/intechopen.72816

National Institutes of Health. (2023). Ashwagandha: Is it helpful for stress, anxiety, or sleep? [Online] Retrieved from: https://ods.od.nih.gov/factsheets/Ashwagandha-HealthProfessional/

Nicolussi, S., Ardjomand-Woelkart, K., Stange, R., Gancitano, G., Klein, P., & Ogal, M. (2022). Echinacea as a potential force against coronavirus infections? A mini-review of randomized controlled trials in adults and children. *Microorganisms, 10*(2), 211. https://doi.org/10.3390/microorganisms10020211

Nicolussi, S., Ardjomand-Woelkart, K., Stange, R., Gancitano, G., Klein, P., & Ogal, M. (2022). Echinacea as a potential force against coronavirus infections? A mini-review of randomized controlled trials in adults and children. *Microorganisms, 10*(2), 211. https://doi.org/10.3390/microorganisms10020211

Ozioma, E. O., & Chinwe, A. N. O. (2019). Herbal medicines in African traditional medicine. *IntechOpen*. https://doi.org/10.5772/intechopen.80348

Ozioma, E. O., & Chinwe, A. N. O. (2019). Herbal medicines in African traditional medicine. *IntechOpen*. https://doi.org/10.5772/intechopen.80348

Passalacqua, N., Guarrera, P., & De Fine, G. (2007). Contribution to the knowledge of the folk plant medicine in Calabria region (southern Italy). *Fitoterapia, 78*, 52-68.

Saggar, S., Mir, P. A., Kumar, N., Chawla, A., Uppal, J., Shilpa, & Kaur, A. (2022). Traditional and herbal medicines: Opportunities and challenges. *Pharmacognosy Research, 14*(2), 107-114.

Saggar, S., Mir, P. A., Kumar, N., Chawla, A., Uppal, J., Shilpa, & Kaur, A. (2022). Traditional and herbal medicines: Opportunities and challenges. *Pharmacognosy Research, 14*(2), 107-114.

Thair, H., Holloway, A. L., Newport, R., & Smith, A. D. (2017). Transcranial direct current stimulation (tDCS): A beginner's guide for design and implementation. *Frontiers in Neuroscience, 11*, 641. https://doi.org/10.3389/fnins.2017.00641

Wachtel-Galor, S., & Benzie, I. F. F. (2011). Herbal medicine. In I. Benzie & S. Wachtel-Galor (Eds.), *Herbal medicine: Biomolecular and clinical aspects* (2nd ed.). CRC Press/Taylor & Francis.

Ward, J. (2023). *History of Native American herbalism: From traditional healing practices to modern applications in medicine and beyond (2023 guide for beginners)*. Barnes & Noble.

Ward, J. (2023). *History of Native American herbalism: From traditional healing practices to modern applications in medicine and beyond (2023 guide for beginners)*. Barnes & Noble.

WHO. (2013). The WHO Traditional Medicine (TM) Strategy 2014–2023 World Health Organization. [Online] Retrieved from: https://iris.who.int/bitstream/handle/10665/92455/9789241506090_eng.pd?sequence=1

WHO. (2023). Integrating traditional medicine in health care. World Health Organization [Online] Retrieved from: https://www.who.int/southeastasia/news/feature-stories/detail/integrating-traditional-medicine

Made in United States
North Haven, CT
05 July 2024

54404998R00102